Health in old age

RETHINKING AGEING SERIES

Series editor: Brian Gearing
School of Health and Social Welfare
The Open University

The rapid growth in ageing populations in Britain and other countries has led to a dramatic increase in academic and professional interest in the subject. Over the past decade this has led to the publication of many research studies which have stimulated new ideas and fresh approaches to understanding old age. At the same time, there has been concern about continued neglect of ageing and old age in the education and professional training of most workers in health and social services, and about inadequate dissemination of the new information and ideas about ageing to a wider public.

This series aims to fill a gap in the market for accessible, up-to-date studies of important issues in ageing. Each book will focus on a topic of current concern addressing two fundamental questions: what is known about this topic? And what are the policy, service and practice implications of our knowledge? Authors will be encouraged to develop their own ideas, drawing on case material, and their own research, professional or personal experience. The books will be interdisciplinary, and written in clear, non-technical language which will appeal to a broad range of students, academics and professionals with a common interest in ageing and age care.

Current and forthcoming titles
Simon Biggs, Chris Phillipson and Paul Kingston: **Elder abuse in perspective**
Ken Blakemore and Margaret Boneham: **Age, race and ethnicity: A comparative approach**
Joanna Bornat (ed.): **Reminiscence reviewed: Evaluations, achievements, perspectives**
Joanna Bornat and Maureen Cooper: **Older learners**
Bill Bytheway: **Ageism**
Beverley Hughes: **Older people and community care: Critical theory and practice**
Anne Jamieson: **Comparing policies of care for older people**
Eric Midwinter: **Pensioned off: Retirement and income explained**
Sheila Peace, Leonie Kellaher and Dianne Willcocks: **Re-evaluating residential care**
Moyra Sidell: **Health in old age: Myth, mystery and management**
Andrew Sixsmith: **Quality of life: Rethinking well-being in old age**
Robert Slater: **The psychology of growing old**
Alan Walker and Tony Maltby: **Ageing Europe**

Health in old age
Myth, mystery and management

MOYRA SIDELL

OPEN UNIVERSITY PRESS
Buckingham · Philadelphia

Open University Press
Celtic Court
22 Ballmoor
Buckingham
MK18 1XW

and
1900 Frost Road, Suite 101
Bristol, PA 19007, USA

First published 1995
Reprinted 1998

Copyright © Moyra Sidell 1995

All rights reserved. Except for the quotation of short passages for the purpose of criticism and review, no part of this publication may be reproduced, stored in a retrieval system, or transmitted, in any form or by any means, electronic, mechanical, photocopying, recording or otherwise, without the prior written permission of the publisher or a licence from the Copyright Licensing Agency Limited. Details of such licences (for reprographic reproduction) may be obtained from the Copyright Licensing Agency Ltd of 90 Tottenham Court Road, London, W1P 9HE.

A catalogue record of this book is available from the British Library

ISBN 0 335 19136 3 (pb)   0 335 19336 6 (hb)

Library of Congress Cataloging-in-Publication Data
Sidell, Moyra, 1940–
  Health in old age: myth, mystery, and management/Moyra Sidell.
    p. cm. – (Rethinking ageing series)
  Includes bibliographical references and index.
  ISBN 0-335-19336-6. – ISBN 0-355-19136-3 (pbk.)
  1. Aged – Health and hygiene. 2. Aged – Health and hygiene – Government policy. 3. Aged – Attitudes. 4. Aged – Health and hygiene – Great Britain. 5. Aged – Health and hygiene - Government policy – Great Britain. I. Title. II. Series.
RA564.8.S55   1994
613´.0438–dc20   94–3589
                                                                                                    CIP

Typeset by Type Study, Scarborough
Printed in Great Britain by Biddles Ltd, Guildford and King's Lynn

Contents

List of tables and figures	vii
Series editor's preface	ix
Acknowledgements	xiii
Introduction	xv

Part I   The health context — 1
1 The mirage of health — 3
2 Lay logic — 18
3 Patterns of health and illness among older people — 33

Part II   Experiencing health — 55
4 Understanding chronic illness and disability — 57
5 Maintaining health with physical illness and functional disability — 70
6 Maintaining health with mental malaise — 90

Part III   Resources for health — 109
7 Health care and the management of health — 111
8 Personal resources and social support — 130
9 A healthy future for old age — 148

Bibliography — 164
Index — 176

List of tables and figures

Figure 0.1	Rectangular survival curve.	xv
Figure 1.1	Suitable domains for assessment of elderly people	9
Figure 2.1	Percentage of men and women who say they do things to keep healthy	23
Table 2.1	Percentage who engaged in health promoting activities	24
Table 2.2	Type of activity engaged in	24
Table 2.3	Explanations of health	28
Table 3.1	Standardized mortality ratios of males in Great Britain	34
Table 3.2	Summary of main findings on immigrant mortality study in England and Wales, 1970–78	34
Figure 3.1	Death rates since 1841 over 65 years	36
Figure 3.2	Life expectancy in selected countries at age 65 and at birth, 1985	37
Table 3.3	Death rate per thousand population for men and women over 55, by age group, England and Wales, 1971–89	38
Figure 3.3	Major causes of death	39
Figure 3.4	Acute sickness in population of Great Britain, 1991	41
Figure 3.5	Accidents, injury and poisoning: All discharges and deaths	42
Figure 3.6	Accidents, injury and poisoning: Consultations to GPs	42
Figure 3.7	Long standing illness in population of Great Britain, 1990	43
Figure 3.8	Limiting long standing illness in population of Great Britain, 1990	43
Figure 3.9	Disability and chronic illness prevalence by age in population aged 65+, 1988	44
Table 3.4	Long standing illness or disability by age groups	44

viii List of tables and figures

Table 3.5	Older respondents with a long standing illness or disability	46
Figure 3.10	Admissions to mental illness hospitals 1986: All diagnoses	47
Figure 3.11	First admissions to mental illness hospitals: Diagnostic group	48
Figure 3.12	Mental disorders: Consultations to GPs	49
Table 3.6	Prevalence reported during the past month of selected mental symptoms in the population over 65 in Great Britain	50
Table 3.7	Prevalence reported during the past month of selected physical symptoms in the population over 65 in Great Britain	50
Table 3.8	Self-assessment of health	52
Table 3.9	Long standing illness or disability by self-assessed health	53
Figure 5.1	The health-ease-dis-ease continuum: Objective and subjective assessments	86
Table 7.1	Estimated programme budget for health care services in England, 1986–87	118
Table 7.2	NHS estimated annual expenditure per head by age group in England, 1986–87	118
Figure 7.1	In-patient admissions in previous 12 months in Great Britain, 1987	119
Table 7.3	Levels of satisfaction with the NHS (per cent) in Great Britain, 1987	120
Figure 7.2	Consultations with GPs	121
Table 7.4	Patients consulting per cent of persons present for the whole of the study year (age groups by frequency of consultation)	122
Table 7.5	Percentage who had consulted their doctor in the two weeks before the interviews	123
Figure 8.1	Self-assessed health: Percentage without good health, by access to material resources, elderly men and women	134
Figure 9.1	Robertson's vision for health	149
Table 9.1	Health care spending as a percentage of gross domestic product (GDP) 1985	152

Series editor's preface

The rapid growth in ageing populations in this and other countries has led to a dramatic increase in academic and professional interest in gerontology. Since the mid-1970s, we have seen a steady growth in the publication of British research studies which have attempted to define and describe the characteristics and needs of older people. Equally significant have been the very few theoretical attempts to re-conceptualize what old age means and to explore new ways in which we think about older people (e.g. Johnson 1976; Townsend 1981; Walker 1981). These two broad approaches which can be found in the literature on ageing – the descriptive (what do we know about older people) and the theoretical (what do we understand about older people and what does old age mean to them) – can also be found in the small number of postgraduate and professional training courses in gerontology which are principally intended for those who work with older people in the health and social services.

Concurrent with this growth in research and knowledge, however, has been a growing concern about the neglect of ageing and old age in the education and basic training of most workers in the health and social services, and about inadequate dissemination of the new information and ideas about ageing to lay carers and a wider public. There is, therefore, a widening gap between what we now know and understand about ageing and ageing populations and the limited amount of knowledge and information which is readily available and accessible to the growing number of professional and voluntary workers and others who are involved in the care of older people.

The main aim of the 'Rethinking Ageing' series is to fill this gap with books which will focus on a topic of current concern or interest in ageing. These will include elder abuse, health and illness in later life, community care and working with older people. Each book will address two fundamental questions: What is known about this topic and what are the policy and practice implications of this knowledge?

Like other books in this series, *Health in Old Age* rethinks a vitally important aspect of ageing. Moyra Sidell does this by taking a critical, exploratory stance towards something which is usually taken for granted in both gerontological literature and popular discourse: the meaning of health and illness in later life. Her book demonstrates that to question the concept of health, to explore the myths and mystery which surround it, is more than just an academic or abstract endeavour. How we view the concept of health underpins what we know, or what we think we know, about health and this in turn affects health policy and practice. As Moyra Sidell puts it, ways of seeing affect ways of knowing which in turn affect ways of doing.

This book is also notable for presenting a truly multi-dimensional picture of what is currently known about health and illness in later life. Surveys have repeatedly confirmed the importance which older people place on having good health. Sidell makes the point, however, that what older people frequently think of as 'good health' differs markedly from the conception of health which underlies most of the research into health in old age, and which broadly reflects the dominant biomedical model of ageing. Whereas that model typically assesses states of health in terms of the absence or presence of disease, qualitative studies of older people's views of their health commonly present an alternative picture in which 'being healthy' is portrayed as a matter of 'feeling good', of being linked to emotional well-being and the ability to cope with the essential tasks of everyday life. As Sidell reports, such qualitative studies are full of people who maintain an optimistic view of their health despite suffering a chronic illness or disability, a paradox which she explores in this book.

Part of the richness of the book lies in its presentation of the voices of older people who we 'hear' talking about their experiences of health and illness in the context of their past and present lives. Some of these personal accounts implicitly challenge the biomedical view of old age by reflecting alternative social, environmental or holistic models of health. Others partly reflect it whilst also drawing on other explanatory frameworks. By vividly depicting the experience of living with a range of states of health, illness and disability these accounts make us question the extent to which we should rely on the dominant biomedical model as the one and only framework for understanding health in later life. To accept the meaning of health as biologically intrinsic or 'given' would be to ignore the biographical evidence presented in chapters 4, 5 and 6 of this book.

Many of these individual histories of health and illness draw on personal frameworks for assessing what it is to be healthy or unhealthy. Whilst deriving in part from the models of health mentioned above they are closely connected to feelings of life-satisfaction, self-esteem and the need to maintain an overall sense of coherence in one's life. One of the strengths of Sidell's book is that, in presenting alternative ways of seeing health, she does not simply seek simply to replace a biomedical account with a more holistic, social or psychological one. As she says, there has been a long and inconclusive gerontological debate in which different sides have been able to bring in evidence to support their points of view. Instead, Sidell highlights the contradictory and conflicting nature of the quantitative and qualitative evidence which emerges from different perspectives and frameworks and explores the implications of these different ways of seeing for describing health and illness in old age, as well as what they suggest for public policy and other forms of intervention.

There is therefore a welcome eclecticism and rich depth to this book which reflects the author's own multi-dimensional approach as a researcher who has sought to understand gender differences in health in old age through types of investigation and analysis which span the quantitative and qualitative, from very 'hard' large nationally collected data samples through to the 'soft' data of life history interviews with older women and men. In drawing on this knowledge and experience in this book, Moyra Sidell has been able to see health in old age in its full complexity and breadth and to suggest to readers new 'ways of seeing' which should enhance their understanding of this very important subject.

Brian Gearing

Acknowledgements

This book is based on a series of studies that I have carried out over the past ten years which have been concerned with the physical and mental health of older people. These studies have used both qualitative and quantitative research methods in order to combine and contrast an aggregate overall perspective of the health of older people, with more detailed personal views from individual older people. My thanks are due to Professor Graham Fennell, who introduced me both to gerontology and to the potential of qualitative research methods.

The quantitative data has been derived from a number of sources, some published, some from my own analysis of large national data sets. I would like to thank the Office of Population Censuses and Surveys for access to the General Household Survey data and the Health Promotion Research Trust for access to the Health and Lifestyle Survey. Access to both these data was facilitated through the ESRC data archive at the University of Essex.

The qualitative data was dependent on the cooperation and generosity of many older people. I am indebted to them for sharing their stories, wit and wisdom with me and for the sheer pleasure of listening to them. I would like to give a special thanks to Hazel Taylor who not only performed the laborious task of transcribing many hours of tape with great patience and sensitivity but also became involved in and delighted by these stories. I am truly grateful to her for her enthusiasm and encouragement and for the benefit of her insight and understanding.

My thanks are also due to Jocelyn Cornwell who initially designed the research into gender differences in health at older ages and to Professor Malcolm Johnson and the School of Health and Social Welfare at the Open University who funded and encouraged the project.

I have been fortunate in having the support of friends and colleagues at the Open University and my warm thanks are due to Jeanne Katz and Julia Johnson for their careful reading and checking of the manuscript; to Linda Jones (who brought health alive for me) and her perceptive comments on drafts of this book; to Brian Gearing who as series editor has been engaged and supportive throughout the whole process; to Christine Jones who typed much of the manuscript and turned my disorderly discs into orderly files, and finally to Jonathan Ingoldby and the staff at Open University Press who have been a pleasure to work with.

The photographs in this volume come mainly from a young photographer Georgina Ravenscroft whose work I first saw in an exhibition put on by Counsel and Care. Georgina has made a specialty of photographing older people which she does with sensitivity and skill and I thank her for allowing me to use her work.

I would also like to thank the following for permission to use copyright material: The Controller of Her Majesty's Stationary Office for figures, extracts and tables from *Population Trends* 1985 and 1990; from OPCS 1988, *The prevalence of disability among adults*, 1993 General Household Survey; Royal College of Physicians London and the British Geriatric Society (1992) for a figure from *Standardised Assessmemt Scales for Elderly People*; Routledge for a figure from M. Blaxter (1990) *Health and Lifestyles*; Elsevier Science Ltd, The Boulevard, Longford, Kidlington, OX5 1GB, for a figure from S. Arber and J. Ginn (1991) 'Gender and inequalities in later life' which appeared in *Social Science and Medicine*, (26), 1; The King's Fund Centre for a figure from Kaleche *et al.* (1988) *Promoting Health among Elderly People*; and from A. Weale (1988) *Cost and Choice in Health Care*; NAHAT (National Association of Health Authorities and Trusts) for tables from Bosanquet *et al.* (1989) *Will you still love me?*; Penguin for a table from P. Townsend, N. Davidson and M. Whitehead (1988) *Inequalities in Health: The Black Report and the Health Divide*; Open University Press for tables from C. R. Victor (1991) *Health and Healthcare in Later Life*, and Ashgate Publishing for figures from J. Robertson (1985) *Future Work*.

Every effort has been made to trace all copyright holders, but if any have been inadvertently overlooked the publisher will be pleased to make the necessary arrangements at the first possible opportunity.

Introduction

Along with a celebration of increased longevity, or the fact that more people are experiencing a long life, comes a distinct sense of unease about that phase of the life cycle. We have a curious ambivalence towards the idea of senescence. Coni and colleagues (1992) point out that on the one hand we consider longevity a highly desirable feature of a society, a feature of developed and mature societies, but we welcome our own senescence with less enthusiasm and some younger people regard old people with a mixture of pity and irritation. Even the word 'senescence' has a pejorative ring although the verb to senesce means simply to grow old. The word senile which derives from the same root is also synonymous with deterioration and decay. So although increased longevity is welcomed, there is concern about the quality of the extra years. Few would disagree with the aphorism that we need to be concerned less with adding years to life and more with adding life to years. Yet achieving it is much more difficult. Some very basic elements important to the quality of life of older people are good health, a reasonable amount of income, adequate shelter and the love and affection of at least one other human being. This book focuses on one of those basic elements, health, although any discussion of health at any point in the life span must also address the issue of wealth or more specifically the lack of it, and the social support that is available to older people.

The relationship of health to old age is an important but complicated and sometimes confused issue. Myths and mysteries abound and its management for the individual and for society is a matter of concern. Ill-health in old age is a source of deep private trouble; it is also a matter of much public policy debate. In personal terms ill-health can bring many losses; the loss of independence and autonomy, loss of mobility, loss of social connections, loss of dignity and privacy, loss of confidence and self-esteem, and it can be the source of pain and suffering. The links between physical health and life satisfaction have long been made (Palmore and Kivett 1977). Public concern with health in old age has characterized older people as a social problem with attendant resource implications.

Sally MacIntyre (1977), in an historical review of public policy in relation to older people between 1834 and 1976, identified two distinct approaches which have been dominant at different times. One approach she describes as a 'humanitarian perspective'. In this perspective the problem is seen to be one of alleviating the distress and suffering of older people. The other approach she terms as an 'organizational perspective'. Here the 'problem' of old age lies in the burden imposed on the rest of society in caring for the infirm. Solutions in terms of this perspective lie in reducing the social and material costs to the rest of society. Logically these two perspectives are incompatible in terms of their solutions. What is fascinating in Sally MacIntyre's analysis is how she describes attempts to reconcile the tensions in these two approaches at certain points during the period she reviews and its relevance for present day policies, particularly in relation to community care. MacIntyre shows how official literature in the 1950s and 1960s presented community care as a solution to the tensions inherent in these two approaches. Rehabilitation and community care were then seen to be in the interests both of the individual older person and the public purse. The intervening years since she wrote her review have confirmed her view that this optimism was false and contradictions have been exposed, that adequate community care which really does benefit individual older people is not cheap. The humanitarian perspective seems to be rapidly disappearing from present day public policy with demographic arguments focusing the public mind on the need for an organizational approach. By concentrating on numbers and using terms like 'the rising tide' and 'burden of dependency' the individual and her/his experience is lost and the problem becomes 'the elderly' who are blocking hospital beds and devouring resources which could be put to better use.

I want to argue that 'the burden of the elderly' and the organizational approach and for different reasons, the humanitarian approach, are all based on assumptions which are open to question. They are all based on very powerful myths. I am aware that 'myth' is a contentious term to use because it has different meanings for different people. I use the term myth to describe views, opinions, assumptions which are prevalent, powerful and in common usage but whose claim to validity is debatable not because they are untruths or fictions but in so far as they claim to represent 'the' truth. It is the notion of 'the truth' or one truth, an essential truth which is there to be discovered which is questionable. I am claiming that there are many truths about health in old age, some which are complementary, some which are contradictory. They are all versions or accounts for which 'evidence' can be summoned to support their claim to validity. Searching for the truth about health in old age is a dubious exercise. Instead in this book I intend to map out the territory of health in old age by exploring, not exploding, the various myths and mysteries which abound.

One of the major 'myths' to explore is the notion of 'the elderly' as a supposedly homogeneous group of people who share sufficient characteristics to warrant lumping together in spite of obvious differences in gender, class, cultural experience and also in age. Then there is what could be termed the

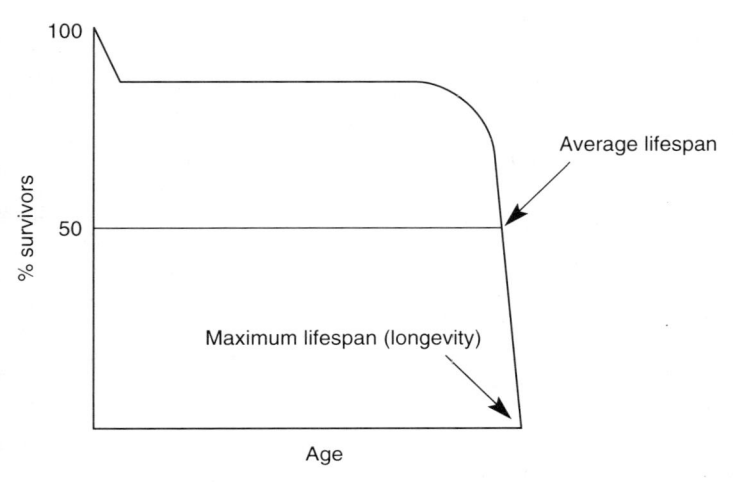

Figure 0.1 Rectangular survival curve

'medical myth', that ageing is synonymous with disease and that any condition that medicine cannot cure is simply 'due to your age'. This can be the cause of a great deal of confusion as Bennett and Ebrahim (1992: 3) point out:

> This association of ageing and disease is the cause of much confusion about what is in store for us as we age, and it is a confusion that tends to affect doctors more than their patients. Patients complain to their doctors of pain and immobility only to be told that their problems are due to their age — which is seldom true.

Evidence to support the 'medical myth' is based on morbidity statistics. These show that diseases are more common among older people than younger people and that the prevalence of chronic illness and disability increases with advanced age. Yet many older people do not suffer chronic illness or disability and many more claim to be in good health in spite of chronic illness.

A competing and seemingly contradictory but more optimistic myth is based on the rectangularization of mortality and compression of morbidity thesis (Fries 1980). This literally graphic account assumes that there is a maximum lifespan for the human species which is approximately 115 years. Greater numbers of people are surviving into their 80s, 90s and 100s which when plotted on a graph draws a near rectangular shape. Deaths are not spread throughout the lifespan but are concentrated in the later years (see fig 0.1).

Fries's thesis is based on the assumption that there is a natural, fixed average lifespan of about 85 years. But this has been challenged on the basis that he has failed to offer any convincing statistical evidence which supports this view (Bytheway 1982). The growing numbers of people living into their second century runs counter to Fries's theory (Bury 1988a). The issue remains highly contentious but has policy implications which will be picked up in Part 3.

Along with the rectangularization of mortality thesis Fries claimed that there is a 'compression' of morbidity, that people are remaining fit, healthy and disease free until a short time before they die. Thus morbidity is compressed into extreme old age. This more optimistic myth does not take account of the potential with increased longevity for accumulating non life-threatening but disabling chronic diseases. And there is evidence that the compression of morbidity myth is more appropriate to the experience of older men than older women (Verbrugge 1984, 1989; Lewis 1985; Sidell 1991; Victor 1991).

An even more optimistic myth which is circulating is what could be termed the 'anti-ageist' myth of the super oldie. The biography section of any bookshop will reveal a number of 'remarkable' 80 and 90 year olds like Charlotte Despard or Bertrand Russell and everyone knows a 'wonderful' old man or woman in their family or living down the road. But although 90 year old marathon runners provide us with more positive images of ageing and a more pleasing prospect than the gloom and doom of disease and decay are they any less oppressive as role models? Are these not unrealistic aspirations based on the evidence of a small number of exceptional individuals? By exploring both negative and positive myths I hope to weave a rich tapestry of problems and possibilities in the territory of health in old age.

As well as the current myths to explore which complicate the picture there are some intriguing mysteries to unravel. One such mystery is that of why, to quote Constance Nathanson (1977), 'women get sick, but men die'. The well documented gender differences in health in old age (Sidell 1991; Victor 1991; Arber and Ginn 1991c) show that women in almost all societies live longer than men but tend to accumulate the more non-life threatening but highly symptomatic conditions as they age. Men who do not die seem to remain more illness free than women. The various reasons which have been offered for this will be explored fully in Chapter 3. Class and ethnic differences in relation to health in old age have received rather less attention than gender differences although Arber and Ginn's recent work on socioeconomic differences in health in later life (1993) provide some insights into the issue of class. Ethnic differences in health in later life is a neglected area of study in terms of large scale sample surveys (Blakemore and Boneham 1993) but insights from small scale studies are beginning to emerge and these will be explored in Chapters 2 and 3.

Another mystery to which there are no obvious answers lies in the question of where responsibility for health lies. If we absorb messages from much of the health promotion literature we would be persuaded to accept the view that we are each individually responsible for our own health. By modifying our behaviour and lifestyles we can affect for good or ill our health chances. That can feel reassuring if we feel in control, firmly in the driving seat. But having responsibility without the information to be in control over our own bodies or the ability to control the wider environment merely induces guilt and gives rise to victim blaming. If, however, we are not responsible for our health then who or what is? Other candidates are the medical profession and the welfare state, but many people resent the interference in their lives. Responsibility for health in old age is particularly difficult to ascribe because health chances will have been set by the cumulative effects of a lifetime. These issues of responsibility for health are bound up with the issue of manageability of health and will be addressed fully in Part 3.

Numerous surveys in both Britain and the USA have found that older people are an anomalous group in that they consistently rate their own health as good in questions designed to elicit a self-assessment of health, when in objective terms, i.e. from morbidity data, their health is shown to be poor. This mystery will be addressed throughout Part 1 but it mostly hinges on perhaps the greatest mystery of all which lies in the concept of health itself. Before we can begin to explore the myths and mysteries that make up the issues of health in old age we need to explore what it is that we mean by health. So much of what we know or think we know about health at all ages depends on how we view the concept of health. 'Ways of seeing' affect 'ways of knowing' and health is a much contested concept. It is a contest in which the medical model of health has dominated in western societies for the last century. But other voices for health are being raised which challenge the dominance of the medical model. Community groups and lay voices are increasingly putting forward social and holistic models of health (Beattie, Jones and Sidell 1992).

The book is divided into three parts. The first part looks at the terms on which we can know about the health of older people and the evidence which is available. The second part looks at older people's experience of health and illness. The third part examines the resources available to people to maintain health at older ages and the implications for public policy.

In Chapter 1 I will explore the various ways of explaining health and relate these different 'ways of seeing' to the way we come to know about and measure health and decide what counts as evidence. These different perspectives have implications for practice and consequently affect 'ways of doing'. I will argue that all these perspectives, even a more holistic account of health, pay more attention to ill-health than to health in a more positive sense. Aaron Antonovsky (1984) claims that we are still dominated by what he calls a 'pathogenic paradigm' in much of our thinking about health and he suggests we should adopt a 'salutogenic paradigm' which will enable us to explore health in a more positive way. Chapter 1 will conclude with a discussion of Antonovsky's thesis and suggest that it offers a useful framework for understanding the health of older people.

Whereas Chapter 1 concentrates on more official and professional accounts of health Chapter 2 focuses on the health beliefs and attitudes of lay people and in particular the ways in which older people explain concepts such as health, illness and disease. The causes older people attribute to ill-health will be explored and how they try to understand and make sense of their own health experiences.

Chapter 3 will examine both the objective and subjective evidence at our disposal for analysing the health status of older people

Part 2 will focus on the experience of health and illness. Chapter 4 will review the theoretical understandings which have been put forward for the way chronic illness and disability affects people's perceptions of their own health and their health choices. This chapter will explore the rationale of a framework for analysing how individuals cope with physical and mental illness and attempt to maintain positive health. This framework will be used to analyse a range of detailed case studies which will be the subject of Chapters 5 and 6.

Part 3 will concentrate on resource and policy implications. Chapter 7 will focus on the health care available to older people and review current policy and provision. Chapter 8 will look at the personal resources at the disposal of older people and the social support available to manage their health. Chapter 9 will review the policy options for a healthy future for old age. It will link back to Chapter 1 looking at the implications for older people of adopting models of health other than the biomedical thus putting health on wider social and political agendas.

PART I

The health context

1

The mirage of health

Introduction

The mystery of why older people consistently rate their health as good when other evidence suggests that the health of older people is not so good can best be explained by reference to another mystery. This is one which relates to the concept of health itself, we therefore need to ask what we mean when we talk of health?

Health is a term we all use and about which we assume that we have a shared understanding, but we might find it hard to define and to agree a definition with others. Researchers into lay health beliefs show that definitions of health vary not only in terms of gender, class and ethnicity but that individuals are not necessarily consistent in their own explanations of health and illness (Stainton-Rogers 1991, Blaxter 1990, Calnan 1987; Cornwell 1984). They may use different explanations depending on their current circumstances and their definitions might change through the life cycle. What research has shown is that people draw on a mixture of official and 'folk' accounts to weave their own explanations of health (Cornwell 1984; Stainton-Rogers 1991). Before going on to look at how older people explain health and illness in Chapter 2, this chapter will explore the repertoire of accounts of health that people have at their disposal to draw on. It will then go on to examine how these different perspectives on health or 'ways of seeing' affect 'ways of knowing' and consequently the measurement of health.

Accounting for health

Accounts of health range from the narrow biomedical account of health as the absence of disease to a very broad, all encompassing 'holistic' account which echoes the World Health Organization definition of health as *a state of complete physical, social and mental well-being* (WHO 1985). As Mildred Blaxter points out this 'has the danger of subsuming all human life and happiness under the label' (Blaxter 1990: 3). Between these two extremes we can identify other accounts which have salience for people such as the environmental account and the biographical account. Although the biomedical account has been dominant in western societies there are signs that we are moving into a phase where pluralism in health accounts is the case, where accounts coexist in a state described by Stainton-Rogers as 'sympatricity', when theories 'operate in parallel, at one and the same time competing and coexisting' (1991: 7).

Biomedicine is still influential in Western societies, with health seen as the absence of diagnosed disease. This view of health is both sanctioned and supported by the health care system. Biomedical explanations relate to the physical body and health is explained in terms of biology. It is a mechanistic view which concentrates on the structure of the body, its anatomy, and the way it works, its physiology. Each body is essentially alike and so health is related to normality, there is a normal structure to the body and a normal way of working. Deviation from these norms represents pathology or a diseased state. This functional view of health sees the human being as a complex organism which can be best understood by breaking it into isolated parts, each with a 'normal' way of working. Disease can then be narrowed down to the malfunction of a particular part of the body. Medical treatment focuses on the diseased part and the tendency is to concentrate on discrete parts or organs and pay less attention to the whole or the interaction of the parts.

This mechanistic and disease orientated view of health inevitably paints a bleak and negative view of the prospects for health in old age. Later life is portrayed as a time of declining strength and increased frailty as organs and tissues wear out or succumb to disease and degeneration. It views individuals narrowly in terms of their bodies which are in decline as the natural consequence of growing older. Hope for better health in old age will come from maintaining the body in better shape, eradicating the diseases to which the ageing body is prone and replacing defective organs. Increasingly medicine is accepting wider social and psychological influences on health and reflecting elements of other models of health. But most doctors and research scientists still believe that the way our bodies work can be understood within a biological framework and that a cause and therefore a treatment can be found for all disorders, even mental disorders.

Biomedicine with its emphasis on the functioning of individual bodies has little to say about emotional and psychological health and some strands of biomedicine have tended to see mental illness as some form of malfunctioning of the brain. Yet the separation of mind and body in explanations of health is a fairly recent phenomenon. In earlier historical periods in western society and in some contemporary eastern cultures mental and physical health are inseparably linked.

Non-biological explanations of health developed separately in western society. Freud explored the role of the unconscious mind in shaping the mental health of the individual. Psychoanalytic theory sees the resolution of unconscious conflicts as essential to mental health. Mental ill-health is then the result of repressing or leaving these conflicts unresolved. Erikson (1965), in his

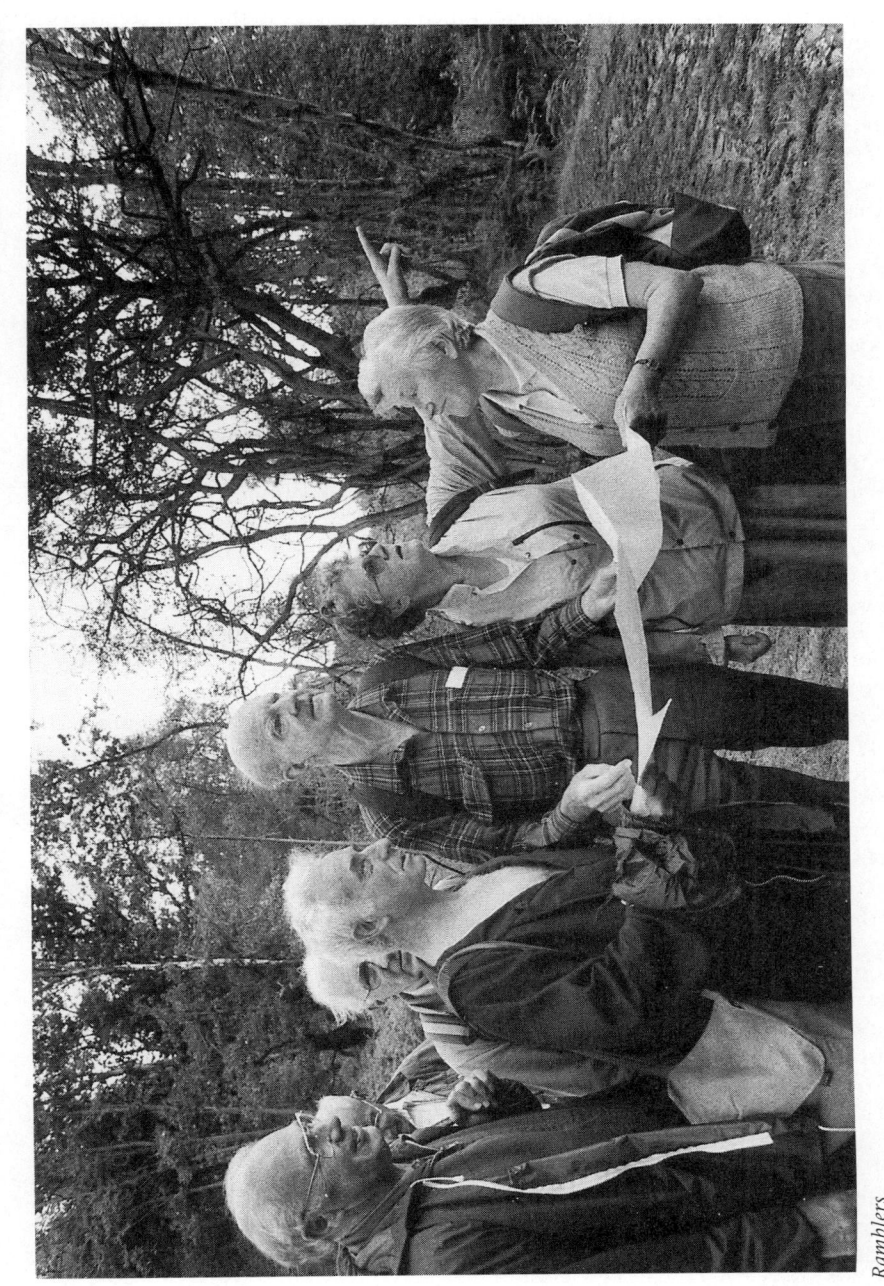

Ramblers
Photograph: Georgina Ravenscroft

revision of Freudian theory, developed notions of a 'healthy personality'. Erikson has been particularly influential in gerontology in that he extended the developmental approach into later life. He identified eight stages of growth from birth to maturity each with a list of traits which indicated 'healthy' or 'pathological' personality patterns and a list of tasks to be fulfilled in order to reach each stage of development. The task of the last stage of life is to achieve 'ego integrity' when one's life has meaning and order resulting in an 'acceptance of one's one and only life cycle as something that had to be and that, by necessity, permitted of no substitutions' (Erikson 1965: 260). The notion of a healthy personality has been further developed by 'humanistic psychology' with an ideal of a healthy person as a thinking, feeling and reflecting being able to change and grow – a rounded, balanced personality (Stevens 1990). Maslow has explored more positive aspects of psychological health with an ideal of health moving from fulfilling basic human needs to reaching a state of 'self-actualization' or 'becoming what one is capable of becoming' (Maslow 1954). In this model self-esteem and the ability to express one's emotions are important elements of healthy growth in people.

A biographical explanation of health (Beattie 1993) has much in common with the humanistic psychology tradition. This account explains a person's health in terms of their biography or the product of their life story and has very clear methodological implications for understanding the health and health needs of older people, which will be explored later in this chapter. The biographic explanation and humanistic psychology are concerned with the whole person and are part of a holistic account of health which emphasizes the person as a unique individual. The older person is not seen as a collection of bodily ills but as a thinking, feeling, creative being who has strengths and weaknesses of body, mind and spirit. It is possible to be healthy in mind and spirit even though the body may be frail. Holism is often linked with equilibrium or a state in which bodies, minds and spirits are in harmony. These are concepts drawn from ancient eastern traditions and have become very popular in the West, particularly in the alternative health movement. But as with biomedicine the focus of attention is on the individual. Critics of a holistic account of health argue that this ignores the impact on the individual of the wider physical and social environment

An environmental or ecological explanation of health has had equally as long a tradition as the biomedical or holistic account but its influence has waxed and waned. The central thinking behind this explanation is that health and disease arise from the relationship of people with both the natural and artificial environment. To promote the health of the population it is necessary to modify or transform that environment. Intervening in the environment has a long history going back centuries to the Romans and ancient Arabic traditions of sewerage, refuge disposal systems and baths (Cipolla 1973; Riley 1987). All these public health measures predated Britain's own Victorian Public Health Movement and the work of Edwin Chadwick (1842). Ironically, although the environmental concerns and the Public Health movement played an important part in the social and political campaigns which led to the creation of the welfare state, the setting up of the National Health Service led to a decline in the influence of public health thinking. The NHS put much of its resources into hospital and primary care and concentrated on treating health problems on an individual basis.

In recent years the environmental account has re-emerged with the realization that biomedicine and the focus on the individual body has not reduced social inequalities in relation to health and disease (Townsend and Davidson 1986; Whitehead 1987). Researchers such as Rene Dubos (1971) and Marc Lalonde (1974) have again drawn attention to environmental causes of health and disease particularly in the economic and social environment.

There is now widespread support for a more overarching social model of health which extends the medical model and draws attention to the adverse effects on health in the physical and social environment, such as poor housing, poverty, pollution, unemployment and poor working conditions (Beattie, Jones and Sidell 1992). This represents a challenge to orthodox medical views and puts health concerns on wider agendas, emphasizing the link between the economic, political and social environment and health.

The social model of health puts less emphasis on decline and decay of the organism and more on the interactions with the physical and social environment. So disease and decline are not inevitable in old age and not attributable to age *per se* but to the conditions in which people age and in which they have lived their lives. Disease is not just 'due to your age' but involves hostile forces in the environment such as poverty and poor housing.

Although the medical model of health has been, and still is, very influential, the new and new-old explanations are being heard and are in turn influencing the medical model. This state of 'sympatricity' is also reflected in research on lay explanations of health and illness with evidence to show that lay people draw on the full range of health explanations at their disposal depending on their situation.

If we accept that there are many meanings of health then we are some way to unravelling the mystery of why older people rate their own health as good when other evidence indicates a high level of pathology. If they see health as more than the absence of disease, if they are drawing on a more holistic or psychological account of health, one which relates more to their self-esteem or degree of life satisfaction then this may be good in spite of suffering from some form of chronic illness or disability. Clearly chronic illness can have a devastating effect on self-esteem and life satisfaction but there is no necessary connection. It is possible to suffer from chronic illness and disability and still 'feel good'. In Chapters 4, 5 and 6 we will develop the interactions between chronic illness disability and psychological well-being. Here I want to argue that the anomaly of older people assessing their health as good in the face of contradictory evidence relates to the kind of evidence that is required to support any one particular explanation of health. Different 'ways of seeing' demand different 'ways of knowing'. What counts as evidence is different if we take a biomedical explanation of health from that required to support a 'holistic' explanation of health. What we 'know' about the health of older people might well be different depending on the perspective we hold on health. What are these different ways of knowing and measuring health?

Measuring health

If we then accept that there are multiple accounts of or ways of seeing health then we also have to accept that there are different ways of measuring health depending on the perception taken. As Alan Beattie points out,

> it is not surprising that often the conflict and competition between accounts of health reflects disputes that are basically epistemological in origin – they revolve around differences of view about what counts as 'reliable' or 'true' knowledge.
>
> (Beattie 1993: 261)

Biomedicine has a well defined and long tradition in measuring health. It is based on the principles of scientific enquiry falling within the philosophical tradition of positivism. This tradition uses mainly quantitative research techniques such as statistical surveys or laboratory experiments. It produces data which is considered 'hard', such as mortality and morbidity statistics or biochemical data such as haemoglobin levels. The focus of attention is not on the person but on the disease or organ which is not functioning normally.

Clearly this type of evidence would not satisfy those whose definition of health is based on a more 'holistic' approach. They would argue that people cannot be viewed as 'mechanical' but must be seen as complex, active and creative individuals. This view puts the human subject at the centre of the research enquiry in an endeavour to describe the 'reality' of people's lives taking into account their wider social and physical environment. This method of enquiry is best described as 'humanistic and qualitative'. It falls within the philosophical tradition of phenomenology which values knowledge that is based on direct experience and attempts to seek out the meaning behind social action. The methods used in these types of enquiry are usually case study and in depth interviewing techniques, for example biographical interviews (Gearing and Dant 1990). The aim of such interviews is to determine the individual's subjective account of his/her health in the context of his/her whole life story. Such data is often referred to as 'soft' because it is always open to interpretation.

A great deal of controversy and debate surrounds the status of these two types of evidence which is not relevant to this book. What we need to acknowledge is that they measure different sorts of health. Mortality and morbidity data will tell us little about whole individuals. However if we hold a medical model of health then we may be less interested in someone's life history or emotional state. In fact most of the evidence we have on 'health' is based on the medical model. Even when a wider account of health is acknowledged, mortality data have to be used in the absence of any other available data. The WHO definition of a more positive view of health as 'a state of complete physical, mental and social well-being' has been widely accepted, but as Nicky Hart observes,

> how can these different dimensions be converted into a measure which can be used to study the distribution of health in one society or to compare standards of health between societies? In the absence of any universally

valid measure, most surveys of health rely on one or other of the health status indicators of morbidity and mortality.

(Hart 1985: 3)

Unfortunately in-depth interviews and life history types of data used in qualitative methodology are not suitable for large scale enquiries and so are not very useful in describing large populations. The Black Report (Townsend and Davidson 1986) which emphasized that health was more than the absence of disease could only base the investigation of inequalities in health on death rates and the prevalence of disease.

An environmental account of health requires evidence of the effects of the physical and social environment on the health of people. It therefore uses measurements of the distribution or incidence of disease in human populations in relation to an element of the physical or social environment. For example in measuring the impact of housing on the health of people, morbidity and mortality is measured in terms of housing tenure to determine if those in poorer rented housing suffer poorer health than those in owner occupied housing. This social epidemiological approach is also in the positivist tradition and is abstract and quantitative. But the focus of attention is the socioeconomic environment and so it is broader than a measurement based on physical health alone.

Ironically attempts to operationalize and measure health in a wider sense have found it necessary to break it down into manageable parts, measuring separately physical, mental, social, economic and environmental factors. For instance, the report of joint workshops of the Research Unit of the Royal College of Physicians and the British Geriatric Society endorsed the various domains which the WHO recommended as appropriate to assessing the health of older people. These domains are shown in Figure 1.1.

The aim of the joint workshop was to recommend standardized scales for measuring each of these domains. Ann Bowling (1991) has pointed out that whilst separate scales have been developed to measure the various elements of a 'holistic' explanation of health such as morale, well-being, functional ability, life-satisfaction and so on 'attempts to combine them have been less successful'. Bowling also points out that a conflict exists between researchers and policy makers in relation to the definition and measurement of health. Policy makers desire straightforward, quantitative measures of health which can be used in decision making. Researchers, mindful of the complexity of the concept of health are more inclined to qualitative measures of health. As she says:

> Researchers are increasingly inclining towards self-ratings of present health; personal evaluation of physical condition; feelings of anxiety, nerves, depression; feelings of general positive affect; and future expectations about health. On the other hand, policy makers may prefer more explicit indicators in their formation of health policy.
>
> (Bowling 1991: 110)

Measuring health, fascinating though it may be, is not an end in itself, nor is it a purely academic exercise. It has a purpose or purposes. It provides essential

> **Activities of daily living** (ADL)
> - physical activities of ADL, i.e. maintaining basic self-care
> - mobility
> - instrumental activities of ADL, i.e. being a functioning member of society and coping with domestic tasks
>
> **Mental health functioning**
> - cognitive
> - presence of psychiatric symptoms
>
> **Psychosocial functioning**
> - emotional well-being in a social and cultural context
>
> **Physical health functioning**
> - self-perceived health status
> - physical symptoms and diagnosed conditions
> - health service utilization
> - activity levels and measures of incapacity
>
> **Social resources**
> - accessibility of family, friends and a familiar/professional, voluntary helper
> - availability of these resources where needed
>
> **Economic resources**
> - income as compared to an external standard
>
> **Environmental resources**
> - adequate and affordable housing
> - siting of housing in relation to transport, shopping and public services

Figure 1.1 Suitable domains for assessment of elderly people
Source: Standardised Assessment Scales for Elderly People, Royal College of Physicians and British Geriatrics Society (1992).

information for the planning of services and the allocation of resources, determining appropriate activities of care such as whether to screen or not to screen for certain conditions. And health measurement is used in the assessment of the outcome of these decisions. In fact measurement or ways of knowing is inextricably linked to ways of doing, i.e. health care. So just as measurement and what counts as evidence is closely related to ways of seeing or perspectives on health, so health care, or the 'doing' of health is also dependent on perspectives of health.

Caring for health

By far the most powerful and some would argue the most successful model of providing health care is the biomedical model. The NHS in Britain is based on this model and has had considerable results in increasing longevity and eradicating disease. The primary goal of biomedicine is to treat and cure disease. The disease has first to be detected in order to apply the appropriate treatment. This is done by a professionally qualified medical practitioner who records the signs and symptoms. Although doctors are now more inclined to listen to the patient's own feelings and versions of their condition, traditionally this has been less regarded than the more 'objective' signs derived from a physical examination or clinical test such as a blood test or X-ray. Nicky Hart summarized the distinctive features of current medical practice as follows:

1. A dominant concern with the organic appearances of disease combined with a tendency to ignore, if not dismiss, the link between mind and body, between physical and mental well-being . . .
2. An orientation towards cure, towards the manipulation of organic symptoms with the intention of effecting their disappearance if at all possible . . .
3. A perception of disease as an autonomous and potentially manageable entity which threatens personal health in temporary or episodic fashion . . .
4. A focus on the isolated individual as the site of disease and the appropriate object of treatment.
5. A belief that the most appropriate place for treatment is a medical environment, the consulting room or the hospital, not the environment where symptoms arise.

(Hart 1985: 11,12)

To today's generation of older people in Britain the universal provision of free medical care at the point of need represented a huge step forward and, for many, a great political victory. Although subsequent generations have come to take this for granted, any erosion of the principles underlying the NHS are immediately challenged. However, Ashton and Seymour (1993) argue that the therapeutic model had its heyday from the 1930s to the 1970s and has since come in for a great deal of criticism. The biomedical model of health care is increasingly being challenged. In fact the concept of the NHS was built on the understanding that once the backlog of ill-health was cleared the improvements in health would lead to a lessening in the demand for health care. Clearly this has not happened. Technological innovation in treatment methods and a seemingly limitless demand for medical care has led to escalating costs and a crisis in the health care system. Much of this is thought to stem from the gains made in increasing longevity which have created a population that is ageing. The successes of this longevity, older people, are then blamed for becoming a burden on this system. But how appropriate is this system of care to older people? Preventing premature death and increasing longevity are obvious benefits. But many of the conditions that face people as they age are not amenable to treatment and cure. We will examine the health profile of older people in Chapter 3, where it will become evident that older people, and especially older women, suffer from chronic conditions which can cause a great deal of pain and discomfort but which are not life-threatening. In fact many of these conditions, such as arthritis, thwart the doctors' urge to treat and cure and consequently are attributed to age.

It is perhaps the failure of biomedicine to cope with the needs of an ageing population which has led to a reassessment of the gains made and to be had by focusing on an environmental explanation of health. It has been argued that many of the improvements in health over the past century were due mainly to public health measures such as improvements in sanitation and housing conditions (McKeown 1976). And the persistence of inequalities in health today are attributed to wider socioeconomic conditions (Townsend and Davidson 1986; Whitehead 1987). This resurgence of interest in the social and environmental influences on health has been termed the 'New Public Health Movement' (Ashton and Seymour 1988) which looks for the causes of ill-health in the environment and so ways of doing are concerned with bringing about change in the physical and social environment. Tackling unhealthy working conditions, pollution, as well as poverty and poor housing are all on the New Public Health agenda. The focus is less on the individual and more on the collective experience of the environment.

What is the potential for improving the health of older people in this approach? From the evidence from the Black Report (Townsend and Davidson 1986) and the Health Divide (Whitehead 1987) it is clear that improvements in the material circumstances of older people will lead to health gains as the Black Report states:

> In old age the relationship between income and the capacity to protect personal health is stronger perhaps than at any other time in the life-cycle, and in general it is likely that individuals who are well endowed through generous or index-linked pension schemes will lead the healthiest, the most comfortable and the longest lives after retirement. These material fortunes or misfortunes of old age are closely linked with occupational class during the working life. To have secure employment and an above-average income when one is at work is to be better able to provide for one's retirement. It is in this way that continuity in the distribution of material welfare is sustained, and inequalities in health perpetuated, from the cradle to the grave.
>
> (Townsend and Davidson 1986: 133)

Improvements in the socioeconomic environment of the population will have cumulative effects on future generations of older people as well as improve the lot of the present generation of older people. These are issues which will be taken up in detail in Part 3.

The tendency of biomedicine to focus on parts of the individual rather than the whole has also been recognized by the medical profession and many practitioners are adopting a more 'holistic' approach. This has been more marked in the case of nursing where a whole person approach has radically changed nursing practice (Pearson and Vaughan 1986, Wright 1990). But 'holism' has been predominantly the philosophy and rationale behind 'non-orthodox' treatment, sometimes known as alternative or complementary therapy. Although some forms of alternative therapies such as acupuncture and osteopathy are becoming more acceptable to orthodox medicine, the practitioners of orthodox medicine in Britain have been deeply suspicious of practitioners of alternative therapy. Much of this scepticism is based on what in biomedicine would be seen as a lack of 'hard' evidence of the benefits of these therapies. Alternative therapists counter this argument by pointing out that biomedicine is imposing its own method of scientific proof on alternative therapy which is wholly inappropriate because the goals of the two forms of treatment are different.

What are the goals of alternative therapy and what does it have to offer older people? An holistic approach to health care is geared to the restoration of equilibrium and is concerned not just with a fit body but also with a well mind or spirit. The need to achieve balance and harmony with one's environment is emphasized but in practice most alternative therapies focus on the individual. Fulder (1988) has outlined five basic features of alternative therapies; these are:

1 A full constitutional and biographical history of the individual is taken and treatment is geared to restoring imbalances, defects and destructive patterns by exploring why they have arisen.
2 Barriers between considering the mind, body and spirit are broken down and everything is thought relevant in treatment including attitude, outlook, energy level, posture as well as lifestyle.
3 Therapy is based on a broad definition of health which includes complete physical and mental well-being.
4 They are well suited to treating chronic, psychogenic and organic diseases which requires a degree of individual resistance.
5 All therapies aim to aid self-healing, they are generally harmless and use non-toxic remedies.

What would this approach have to offer older people if it were freely available? Broadly, alternative therapies offer relief from symptoms such as pain and stiffness and they offer an understanding of the effect on health of emotional burdens which many older people carry, such as an accumulation of losses. To heal rather than to cure is the aim, which is particularly relevant to degenerative conditions such as arthritis. Unlike biomedicine which mainly seeks to cure this does not lead to a sense of hopelessness and failure. For older people suffering from chronic and potentially disabling conditions alternative therapies seem to have much to offer. Unfortunately, alternative therapies are not freely available. They remain mainly in the Private Sector, and are therefore financially beyond the reach of the majority of older people. There is also a concern that whilst most practitioners are well qualified and operate with integrity, the present unregulated status of alternative therapies allows for a minority of unscrupulous practitioners to prey upon the vulnerabilities of sick people.

The holistic approach centres on the whole person and that person must be an active participant in the therapy. Advocates of alternative therapy claim that this gives control to the individual. Indeed the holistic approach is premised on the view that responsibility for health lies with the individual. Critics of alternative health see this as potentially 'victim blaming'.

> [Holism] appears to give an individual an unparalleled sense of participating in, perhaps even controlling, his or her own well-being. Yet this profound conviction that lying within each and every one of us is the kernel of a whole person is not without its problems . . . .In the idea of the

whole person, the possibility that an individual has control over health and the possibility that an individual is to be blamed for disease often shade into one another.

(Coward 1989: 68–69)

Having greater control over one's health can be either a liberating or a daunting experience. One of the greatest criticisms of biomedicine is that health care is totally under the control of the medical profession with the role of patient being one of compliance. 'Following doctors orders' without question was for Talcott Parsons (1975) the essence of an ideal patient. However there are new messages coming from biomedicine which are concerned with the prevention of ill-health. These put responsibility for changing unhealthy habits and adopting more healthy lifestyles firmly on to the individual. This appears to give choice and control back to the individual but it can lead to defining ill-health as personal pathology resulting from a chosen lifestyle. It thus becomes a form of 'victim blaming'. Biomedicine and alternative approaches to health care both individualize health.

Just where responsibility for health lies is an important question for older people. Much of the 'panic' about the growing numbers of older people is about the burden this puts on the health care system. If somehow they only have themselves to blame then their 'right' to free health care could well be eroded. In an atmosphere of fierce competition for resources in health care and notions of rationing, older people could well lose out. Clearly everyone would like to feel more in control of their health but we know from the Black Report (Townsend and Davidson 1986) and numerous other studies that much of our ill-health is beyond our individual control and that the remedy lies in the realm of public policy. We require information if we are to take more control of our own health and that is something which the medical profession has, in the past, been loath to share. Information is a precious resource for health and this subject will be returned to in detail in Part 3 where the resource implications of these different models of care will also be discussed.

Much of the discussion so far has been concerned with dealing with ill-health. Even a holistic account of health is often couched in terms of countering the effects of ill-health. All the accounts of health explored so far see the normal state of affairs to be one of homeostasis. Any disruption of this homeostasis is considered abnormal and if homeostasis is not restored then the organism is said to be in a state of pathology or diseased. Aaron Antonovsky (1984) has called this 'the pathogenic paradigm' and he claims that all our models of health are dominated by this paradigm, even the biopsychosocial models.

Antonovsky (1984: 115) draws out some of the consequences of this domination. The first is that 'we have come to think dichotomously about people, classifying them as either healthy or diseased'. Those categorized as 'healthy' are normal, those categorized as non-healthy or diseased are deviant. There is no place in this dichotomy for those who have a chronic illness yet are able to function perfectly well or for those who have a handicap yet are well satisfied with life. Second, and this echoes the holistic account, we have come to think of specific diseases such as cancer or heart disease instead of being in a state of dis-ease. We have become obsessed with morphology instead of theory and practice in relation to generalized dis-ease and its prevention. This leads to Antonovsky's third concern which is that we tend to look for specific causes for these specific diseases in order that the causes can be eradicated instead of accepting that 'pathogens are endemic in human existence' (p. 115). He believes that we need to explore the capacity of human beings for coping with pathogens. Fourth, the pathogenic paradigm deludes us into thinking that if we can eliminate 'disease' we will have health. This 'mirage of health' (Dubos 1961) has been the driving force behind the 'technological fix' and 'magic bullet' attitude to eradicating disease. This attitude leads to the fifth consequence that Antonovsky identified which is that the pathogenic paradigm concentrates on 'the case' or identifies high risk groups instead of studying the 'symptoms of wellness' (p. 116). Adopting this approach would entail studying the smokers who do not get lung cancer or the 'fat eaters' who do not have heart trouble.

Antonovsky believes that we should think 'salutogenically'. He claims that instead of assuming that the normal state of the human organism is one of homeostasis, balance and equilibrium it makes more sense to acknowledge that the 'normal state of affairs for the human organism is one of entropy, of disorder, and of disruption of homeostasis' (1984: 116). He suggests that none of us can be categorized as either healthy or diseased but that we all can be located somewhere along a continuum which he calls 'health-ease-dis-ease'. He explains:

> We are all somewhere between the imaginary poles of total wellness and total illness. Even the fully robust, energetic, symptom-free, richly functioning person has the mark of mortality: he or she wears glasses, has moments of depression, comes down with flu, and may well have as yet non detectable malignant cells. Even the terminal patient's brain and emotions may be fully functional.
>
> (1984: 116)

This way of thinking would have profound effects on the way we view health in old age. It would discourage a percentage approach to assessing the health of older people. Instead of assuming that because 60 per cent have a chronic illness or disability they are therefore in poor health whilst the other 40 per cent are in good health, we would need to look behind those figures to ask how those 60 per cent are actually affected by their chronic illness or disability and to explore their wellness. We would have to ask questions such as why do some people cope whilst others do not, why some consider themselves to be healthy in spite of their chronic illness whilst others do not. We would also need to ask about the dis-ease of the 40 per cent without chronic illness or disability. Do they have non-classifiable aches and pains, discomforts and feelings of unwellness?

Antonovsky is anxious that this reorientation towards health does not minimise the achievements of medical science nor that it should impede the progress of technological change. Rather his purpose is to redress an imbalance inherent in the way we view health, not to abandon the struggle against disease but to widen the armoury and explore other ways of achieving health.

We need the availability of hip replacement surgery but we also need to understand why one person copes well with the operation and fully regains mobility while another does not. We need to identify all the factors which might help us move along the continuum and not just focus on the disease, to ask not so much how we can eradicate certain stressors but how we can learn to live with them, concentrating on the ability to adapt.

When exploring the health of older people Coleman's work on adjustment in later life is relevant to the way people adjust to chronic illness and disability and this will be explored in Chapters 5 and 6. Another feature of the salutogenic paradigm which helps in our understanding of health in later life is that it turns on its head the notion that older people are a high risk group. As Antonovsky says, all of us 'by virtue of being human are in a high risk group' (1984: 117). If we locate people dynamically along a continuum of health then we are less likely to stereotype 'the elderly' as diseased. By adopting a salutogenic paradigm we can reconceptualize questions about health in later life to concentrate on why and how people cope well with chronic illness and disability. The questions change from what stops people becoming sick to what helps them to become healthy in spite of disease.

In an attempt to define the mechanisms which help people to cope with adverse health conditions Antonovsky developed a construct which he calls a *sense of coherence*, abbreviated to SOC. He describes it as follows:

> The sense of coherence is a global orientation that expresses the extent to which one has a pervasive, enduring though dynamic feeling of confidence that one's internal and external environments are predictable and that there is a high probability that things will work out as well as can reasonably be expected.
>
> (Antonovsky 1979: 123)

In a later refinement he identified three main components: comprehensibility, manageability and meaningfulness. Comprehensibility is the ability to see one's own world as understandable, to 'have confidence that sense and order can be made of situations' (1984: 118). One views the future as reasonably predictable rather than chaotic, disordered or unpredictable. Meaningfulness is the 'emotional counterpart of comprehensibility ... life makes sense emotionally' (Antonovsky 1984: 119). Life is worth living for those who see their lives as comprehensible and meaningful. Manageability reflects the extent to which people feel that they have adequate resources, mental, physical, emotional, social and material, to meet whatever demands are put upon them.

Antonovsky is not alone in identifying factors which enable people to cope with difficulties. Brown and Harris (1978) identified 'protective factors' in their study of depression in young women and Murphy (1982) also identified 'confidantes' as a protective factor against depression among older women. Kobasa *et al.* (1981) developed a concept of hardiness which is not dissimilar to Colerick's (1985) concept of stamina in later life and connections obviously can be made to Rotter's 'Health Locus of Control' (1966). However Rotter categorizes people as being either 'internals' or 'externals' that is, they feel that their health is either within their control or beyond their own control and in the hands of powerful others or fate or god. Antonovsky points out the difference with his SOC:

> when people are high on manageability, they have the sense that, aided by their own resources or by those of legitimate others, they will be able to cope and not grieve endlessly. Moreover, there will be no sense of being victimized by events or of being treated unfairly by life.
>
> (1984: 119)

His argument is that wherever a person is located on the health-ease-dis-ease continuum at any particular time those with a stronger SOC are more likely to move towards the health end of the continuum.

A person's SOC is built up from a range of experiences and sources through the life cycle and should be well developed by adulthood. Antonovsky sees the SOC developing from the degree to which our life experiences provide 'consistency', an 'underload/overload balance' and provide for participation in decision making. We experience consistency when a given behaviour results in the same consequences whenever we exhibit it and when people respond to us in consistent ways. This allows us to predict the outcome of behaviour and therefore our lives seem reasonably predictable. Underload/overload balance is achieved when the demands made upon us are appropriate to our capacities. Underused capacity due to lack of challenges can be as harmful as not having sufficient capacity to meet the challenges with which we are faced. The extent to which we participate in decision making is important to the emergence of a strong SOC and is the basis of the meaningfulness component. When everything is decided for us and we have no say in the matter, when the rules are set by others without consultation then the experience is alien to us. The issue is not so much having control over the events of our lives but in having some part in the decision making process.

Antonovsky's notion of a SOC which can predict the way people react to ill-health remains at the level of theorizing; as he points out it has not been put to the test of empiricism, and it is not the purpose of this book to engage in that process in relation to older people. Rather Antonovsky's theory provides a useful framework for analysing the health status of older people both collectively and individually. The health-ease-dis-ease continuum allows us to locate older people along the continuum rather than categorizing them in terms of either health or disease. It allows us to explore how people move along the continuum towards the health end in spite of chronic illness disability or psychological malaise which is the subject matter of Part 2. His SOC provides a framework for analysing the resources available to older people to provide for their health needs in Part 3. But first in the next two chapters of Part 1 we will explore the attitudes and beliefs that older people hold in relation to health and illness and then in Chapter 3 take an overview of the evidence we have on the health status of older people using both subjective qualitative and objective statistical evidence.

2

Lay logic

Introduction

In Chapter 1 we explored a range of explanations of health which could be described as official accounts. They are accounts used by experts, academics and health professionals. Increasingly attention is being given to what lay people say about health and how it affects the quality and meaning of their everyday lives. It is, however, important to bear in mind that the distinction between lay and professional views is very blurred and it would be false to see them as mutually exclusive. Professionals are also lay people and may have personal views which conflict with their professional perspective. And it is clear that lay people frequently draw on official accounts in their own explanations about health and illness.

In this chapter we will explore what we know about older people's explanations of health and illness because it is important to know how people view health in order to understand how people are likely to respond to their own health and illness. Much of the rationale behind the Health and Lifestyles Survey (Cox *et al.* 1987) was to investigate the links between on the one hand attitudes and beliefs about health and illness and on the other health promoting behaviours and illness behaviour, for example, the ways in which people seek help. It is not suggested that older people as a group hold one set of beliefs and attitudes to health and illness or that individuals hold constant and consistent views. But it is useful to explore what we know about the range of views held by older people and to tease out common themes and patterns. In order to set older people's explanations in some context we will first look at the work done on lay perspectives on health and illness across the age range.

Lay perspectives on health and illness

Systematic investigation of lay health beliefs in western societies is a fairly recent phenomenon but the last 20 years has seen a great deal of activity in this area. Studies fall into two categories: those which explore what lay people think constitutes health and those which explore what lay people think causes disease. This latter aspect is particularly important when considering questions about responsibility for health and who or what is to blame for illness.

Claudine Herzlich (1973) was one of the pioneers in the field of investigating lay health beliefs. In the late 1960s she carried out in-depth interviews with predominantly middle class people in France, particularly in Paris and Normandy, to ascertain their beliefs about health and disease. Her work influenced later researchers including those who explored the health beliefs of older people (Blaxter and Paterson 1982; Williams 1990). She identified three main ways in which her respondents conceptualized health:

1 health-in-a-vacuum or health as the absence of disease;
2 health as a reserve – something to be had, a strength and potential to resist illness;
3 health as a state of equilibrium characterized by positive well-being, happiness, feeling strong and getting on well with people.

In the 1980s research into lay accounts of health and illness has been carried out in Britain by Calnan (1987), Blaxter (1983), Cornwell (1984) and Stainton-Rogers (1991). Michael Calnan (1987) in his investigation into the health views of a sample of 60 women in southeast England was keen to explore class differences. He identified four concepts of health.

1 health as never ill;
2 health as being able to get through the day, to carry out routines;
3 health as being fit and active, taking exercise;
4 health as being able to cope with stresses and crises in life.

Calnan found that the working class women were more likely to use the first two explanations of health whereas the middle class women in his study used the last two more frequently. Both Calnan's and Herzlich's studies were relatively small scale and were based on under 100 respondents. Mildred Blaxter has drawn on these in-depth studies and her own study of mothers and daughters (Blaxter and Paterson 1982) to inform the design of the Health and Lifestyles Survey (HLS) which taps the health beliefs and attitudes of a nationally representative sample. This study was able to draw on the views of 9000 respondents and, by using a much more open ended approach to asking questions than is used in most sample surveys, it was able to identify a rich diversity of views about health. Most of the respondents in the HLS expressed more than one definition of health. The following list of the full range of concepts of health used by respondents to the Health and Lifestyles Survey represents those diverse views:

> health as not ill;
> health as absence of disease/health despite disease;
> health as a reserve (strength);

health as behaviour, health as the 'healthy life';
health as physical fitness;
health as energy, vitality;
health as social relationships (relating well to others);
health as function;
health as psycho-social well-being.

Blaxter narrowed the concepts down to four main ones which echo the findings of Calnan and Herzlich. These were: health as the absence of disease, health as physical fitness and energy, health as being functionally able and health as being psychologically fit.

Concepts of illness

In the French study mentioned above Claudine Herzlich (1973) explored with her interviewees their concept of illness. She found that they categorized illness in four ways: serious, possibly fatal illnesses, chronic illnesses, trivial illnesses such as colds and flu and childhood illnesses. From her respondents' replies Herzlich was able to identify three metaphors for illness.

- The illness as destroyer metaphor was held by those who saw illness as curtailing everyday life and social interaction. For them illness was to be avoided or denied.
- The illness as occupation metaphor was held by those who accepted the illness but who strove to fight against it putting all their resources into the fight.
- The illness as liberator metaphor, on the other hand, provided the opportunity to opt out of one's responsibilities and avoid stressful situations to gain sympathy.

Other research into the meaning of illness has explored how 'lay' people perceive the cause of illness and who or what is responsible and therefore to blame for that illness.

Jocelyn Cornwell (1984) carried out in-depth biographical interviews with 24 people living in the East End of London to ascertain their explanations of health and illness. She identified two distinct types of accounts. One she called public, the other private. Public accounts were lay interpretations of official accounts. They would typically be responses to specific questions about health or the cause of illness and they were attempts to give a 'right' answer. Private accounts arose out of personal experience and would be disclosed as part of the conversation rather than as an answer to specific questions. These experiences were, she found, more likely to be recounted when the researcher was more familiar with the interviewee. This has implications for the type of information which can be obtained from sample surveys where the questions are specific and the interviewer has little opportunity to build up a rapport with the interviewee.

Cornwell found that public accounts of illness causation were more linear than private accounts. The cause of illness could be thought of as either internal or external but rarely did her respondents attribute blame to themselves. They were mainly working class and economically disadvantaged people who did not consider they were capable of changing their lifestyles in order to avoid illness. But they did believe that adopting the right attitude to illness was important – not giving in to illness and not being defeated by it. Being a survivor was a moral imperative. More private explanations of illness were extremely complicated and inextricably bound up with their life history. Causation of illness was seen as less linear and had more to do with the interconnectedness of events. Thus attributing blame was not appropriate and they were more engaged with the 'what ifs'. Cornwell saw her respondents' views on health and illness as a product of their 'hard-earned' lives which were characterized by struggle, grit and determination. The issue was more about overcoming illness than avoiding it.

Health behaviours

The willingness of people to engage in disease prevention and health promoting behaviours depends on a range of variables. Age is important but social class has received a great deal of attention. The relationship of social class to preventative health behaviours is one that Pill and Stott (1981, 1982, 1985) have investigated amongst mainly working class people in Wales. They were able to identify both those who felt that they were at the mercy of ill-health and those who felt they had some control over whether they became ill or not. They developed a 'Salience of Lifestyle Index' (SLI) with which they characterized their respondents as either 'fatalists' or 'lifestylists'. Fatalists were low on SLI and saw themselves as powerless and having no personal responsibility for their health. Lifestylists were high on SLI. They believed that by adopting a healthy lifestyle, ill-health could be avoided and so they were more susceptible to health education campaigns. Pill and Stott also found that there were those whose score fell in the middle of the SLI range who saw stupid and careless behaviour as responsible for certain illnesses and considered it one's duty not to indulge in such behaviour but who nevertheless did not feel they were otherwise in control of their health. Much of Pill and Stott's work is concerned with how people are likely to respond to health education campaigns and their SLI is in some ways similar to Rotter's Health Locus of Control (1966) in that it seeks to locate people on a scale of feeling in control of their health. Wendy Stainton-Rogers reviews both of these scales (1992) and concludes that they are very limited in their application. She argues that people use different explanations of health at different times in their lives depending on the circumstances – that they have a range of explanations to draw on which might well conflict. She identifies eight such accounts of health and illness which also have implications for the attribution of blame and responsibility.

1 The 'body as machine' account. This corresponds closely to the medical model. To run smoothly the body needs to be fed and properly maintained. If it breaks down it can be fixed with modern medicine.
2 The 'body under siege' account. In this account the body is consistently besieged by external threat of disease and stressful events which render the individual helpless but not without feelings of guilt and blame.

3 The 'health promotion' account. This is similar to Pill and Stott's 'lifestylists'. Good health was a matter of adopting the right lifestyle and individual health promoting behaviour.
4 The 'inequality of access' account. Here poor health is related to socio-economic inequalities and unfair allocation of resources. This is certainly beyond the individual's sphere of responsibility, and blame is laid at the feet of the government.
5 A 'cultural critique' account. In this account it is less the inequitable allocation of resources but the unequal distribution of power and access to knowledge which determines health.
6 The 'God's power' account. In this account good health is the gift of God and the product of good living.
7 The 'willpower account'. This is a mind over matter account which stresses the self-healing properties of the human organism.
8 The 'robust individualist' account. Here freedom of choice is all important and this includes the freedom to indulge in health risking behaviours. It is the individual's body to use or abuse as he or she pleases.

Accounts 1, 3 and 7 are more likely to encourage the adoption of health promoting behaviours, account 8 could result in either healthy or unhealthy behaviour but it gives choice and a sense of control to the individual. The notion of choice and control are lacking in accounts 2, 4, 5 and 6 and would probably encourage a more fatalistic attitude.

Kathryn Backett and Charlie Davidson have investigated the perception of health and attitudes to health promoting behaviours at different stages of life. Their work is based on two qualitative studies conducted in Edinburgh and south Wales. The stage of life was, they found, an important factor for their respondents in considering what was reasonable health behaviour. So while 'burning the candle at both ends' was an acceptable and even life-enhancing behaviour for young people, it was thought to be inappropriate and damaging to older people. The issue for middle aged and older respondents was whether it was too late to change to the health promoting behaviours currently being urged on people. Many were aware of the damage that had already been done both by the environment and their previous lifestyles. But also as people got older they were less impressed by health education messages, as Backett and Davidson note:

> Their ideas about effective or ineffective healthy behaviours were now strongly grounded in experience; and many were scathing about the faddishness of current healthy ideas. Rather, they extolled ideas which they felt were common-sense, such as paying attention to weather conditions, wearing sensible clothing and treating minor ailments sensibly.
> (Backett and Davidson 1992: 58)

The Health and Lifestyles Survey asked their respondents 'do you do anything to keep yourself healthy?'. The older respondents as much as the younger respondents claimed to engage in activities to keep themselves healthy. Figure 2.1 shows the percentage of men and women who claimed to do so broken down by age groups and social class.

Males   ## Females

[Bar chart showing percentages by age group (18-39, 40-59, 60+) for Non-manual and Manual categories, for Males and Females]

Claims to do things to keep healthy

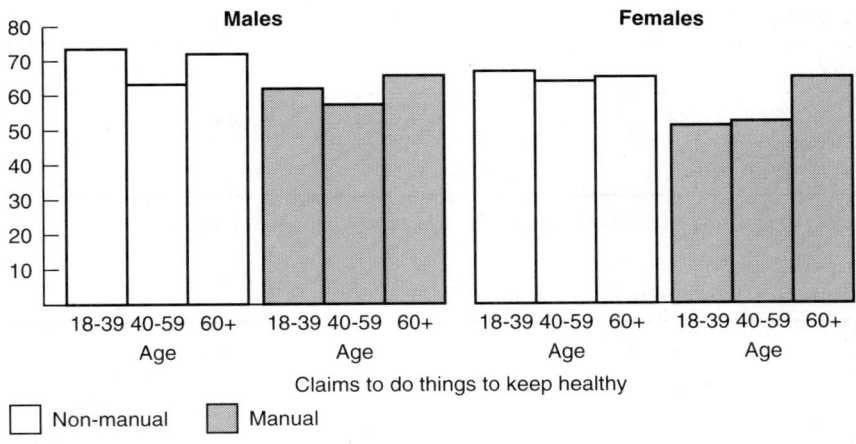

☐ Non-manual   ▨ Manual

Figure 2.1 Percentage of men and women who say they do things to keep healthy.
Source: Blaxter, 1990: 166.

It is the middle age band who claim to engage in less health promoting behaviours with older working class men and women doing more than the younger and middle aged groups. On this evidence there is no indication that older people think it is too late to take part in health promoting behaviours. Rakowski and Hickey claim that it is important to take into account a time perspective in considering the likely health promotion behaviours of older people — that older people are less likely to take on health promoting behaviours if they possess 'constricted future expectations' (Rakowski 1979). They elaborate on this theme:

> Beliefs that the future is unimportant, that one has accomplished all that was intended in life, or that one is living on 'borrowed time' are almost sure to have some impact on health behaviour.
> (Rakowski and Hickey 1980: 287)

Future expectations might be quite different for a 65 year old than they are for an 85 year old. Secondary analysis of the HLS data shows the different levels of health behaviour engaged in by different age groups within the category 'old' (Table 2.1).

There is a 10 per cent drop in health behaviour between the younger old and the older old but the gap between men and women at each of the age groups is greater, about 12 per cent. We can only speculate on the reasons for this gap. Is it because men have greater opportunities for activities than women or is it because women suffer from more chronic and symptomatic conditions than men which might inhibit their ability to engage in health promoting activities? Analysis of the sorts of activities which they engage in throws some light on this. This analysis is shown in Table 2.2.

Men engage in more active pursuits such as gardening, sports and leisure and walking although walking is also a major pursuit of women. Doing one's housework was mentioned more by women and so was a healthy diet. Within

The health context

Table 2.1 Percentage who engaged in health promoting activities

Men			Women		
65–74	75–84	85+	65–74	75–85	85+
n = 448	n = 215	n = 16	n = 592	n = 291	n = 53
73	69	62	61	56	49

Source: Health and Lifestyles Survey 1987; own analysis of unpublished data.

Table 2.2 Type of activity engaged in

	Men (%)			Women (%)		
	65–74	75–84	85+	65–74	75–84	85+
	n = 448	n = 215	n = 16	n = 592	n = 291	n = 53
Walking	34	29	37	23	19	6
Gardening	25	27	35	7	8	4
Healthy diet	12	9	–	20	14	15
Leisure activities	12	11	–	11	6	6
Housework	4	8	6	9	13	9
Social activities	4	6	–	6	6	2
Get fresh air	6	10	6	8	4	2
Sporting activities	7	3	–	3	2	–
Lose weight	2	1	–	3	1	–
Cut down alcohol	3	1	–	1	1	3
Give up smoking	4	1	–	1	–	–

Source: Health and Lifestyles Survey 1987; own analysis of unpublished data.

each category for both men and women the numbers engaging in the activity diminishes with age, although the actual numbers of older men in the over 85 age group are too few from which to generalize. Increasing levels of chronic illness and disability must affect the opportunity to engage in health promoting activities. But the health related activities that older people engage in are very much the everyday accustomed behaviours of a lifetime. What are the health beliefs and attitudes of older people on which these health related behaviours are based?

Concepts of health and illness held by older people

One study which compared two generations of mothers was Blaxter and Patersons' (1982) in-depth qualitative study of working class grandmothers and their daughters. The concept of health used by both mothers and grandmothers was one of being able to function normally, to go about their daily business. Their expectations of health were very low and they did not equate health with a sense of well-being or of achieving a degree of physical fitness. Thus both grandmothers and mothers were reflecting the health norms of their class and neither generation was inclined to indulge in health promoting behaviours other than those to do with carrying on normal activities. In fact they were quite scathing of such practices:

> You'll find a' this health-food fanatics an' keep-fit fanatics nae ony healthier than a person that just does their normal – their normal work, normal meals.
>
> (Blaxter and Paterson 1982: 29)

Disease they thought was outside of their control. The older women put great emphasis on the role of heredity in disease causation. Most diseases were considered to be 'in the family' and as Blaxter and Paterson reflect:

> Since many conditions had in fact repeated themselves through several generations of a poor environment, their reasoning was not illogical, and the appeal to heredity appeared to provide a justification for fatalism.
>
> (ibid.: 36)

When disease was considered to be caused by neglect of themselves they felt they had had no choice in the matter;

> And I had pleurisy, and there wis naebody to look after me, I just used to come an' get my poultice and heat it at the fire and put it back on. I ken whit it wis, it wis really neglect, my own – well, no' my own fault, I had to look efter the bairns, you understand.
>
> (ibid.: 36)

As well as heredity and neglect diseases were also thought to be caused by external environmental agents such as damp, harsh climates and poor working conditions. The younger mothers also considered heredity to be an important factor in the causation of disease but they were less likely to see neglect or environmental factors being quite so important. They considered people to be better off now, as one mother put it, 'There's nobody starving now' (ibid.: 36).

If disease was more or less outside of one's control, as with Cornwell's East-Enders, 'giving in' to illness – the experience of the symptoms of disease – was certainly not. Blaxter and Paterson maintain that for all their respondents, but particularly the older ones, illness was a moral category. They report that this was a constant theme in the interviews. Illness was associated with a lack of moral fibre, it was due to 'imagination' or 'hypochondria' or self-indulgence. Illness could be overcome by strength of character. Understandably most people were therefore reluctant to describe themselves as anything but healthy, given that they held a view of health as the absence of disease and illness.

In Blaxter's later work (1990), based on the much larger survey of people's attitudes and beliefs about health (Cox *et al.* 1987), she noted that those who were themselves in poor health were less likely to express health as not ill. This was very marked amongst the older people in the survey; 22 per cent of men and 16 per cent of women over 60 who were without chronic illness held this explanation of health but only 10 per cent of men and 6 per cent of women who did have a chronic illness used it. This could well explain how those who in 'objective' terms have poor health still describe themselves in reasonably

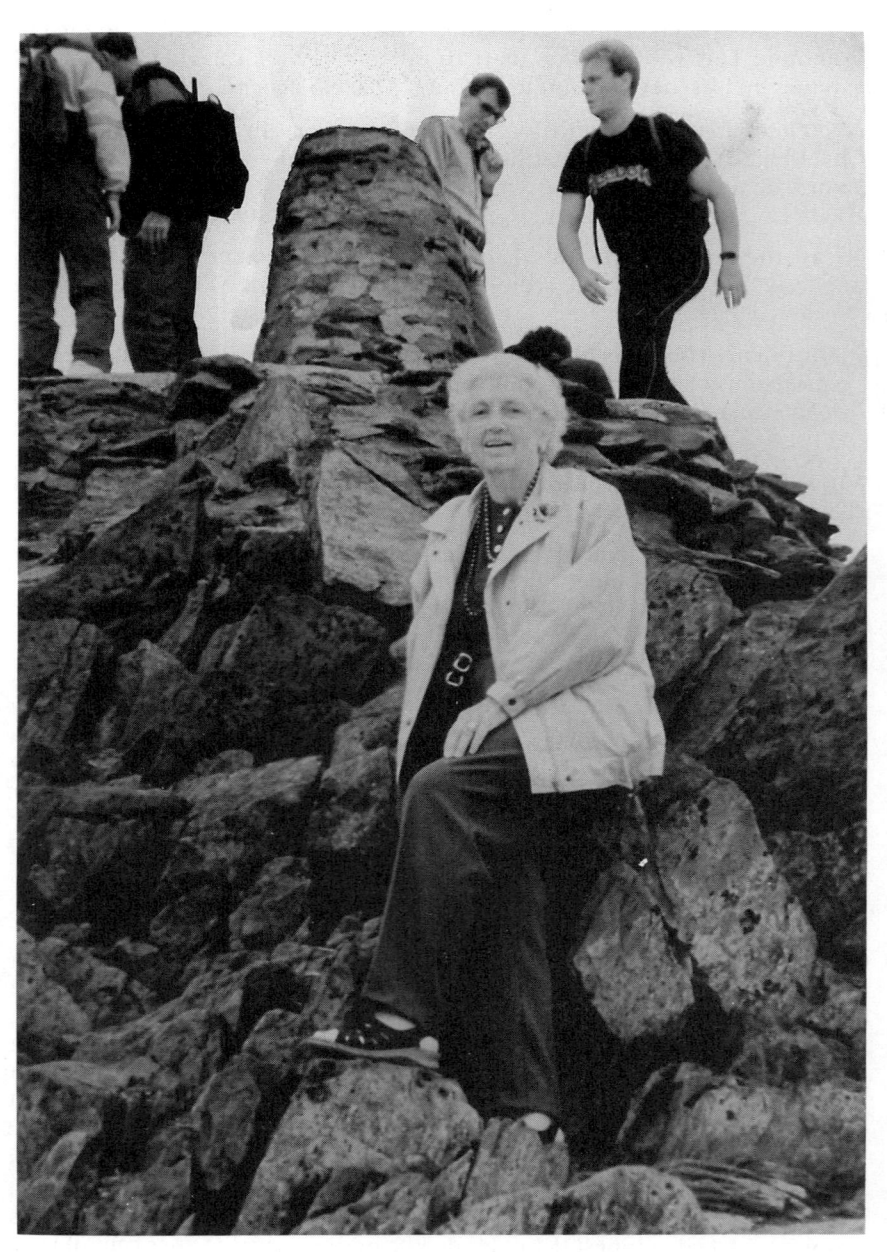

'On top of things'

good health. They are not using health in relation to illness or disease but are more likely to see health as a more psychosocial sense of well-being. Health as physical fitness was also less favoured as an explanation of health with the older respondents to the Health and Lifestyles Survey. But health as energy or vitality was an explanation which was used by many older people, like one 74 year old man who described it in terms of tackling jobs: 'you feel ready to get on with anything that needs doing. You feel that you can tackle any physical work' (Blaxter 1990: 26). For older women this was interpreted as being able to do one's housework and was described as health as functional ability.

Maintaining social relationships and having enough energy to help others was important to older people. A 79 year old woman disabled with arthritis said: 'To be well in health means I feel I can do others a good turn if they need help', and another 74 year old woman said, 'You feel as though everyone is your friend, I enjoy life more, and can work and help other people' (ibid.: 27).

Whereas Blaxter and Paterson's sample of mothers and daughters held a mainly physical and functional view of health and did not see health as a more positive state or a feeling of well-being, this finding was not borne out by the larger HLS where many of the older people as well as the younger people saw health as psychosocial well-being. This explanation was used more frequently by those who had more education which could account for why the working class women in the 1982 study were unlikely to use this explanation. Many older people in the HLS associated health with happiness. One 74 year old farmer's widow described health in very enthusiastic terms:

> I've reached the stage now where I say isn't it lovely and good to be alive, seeing all the lovely leaves on the trees, it's wonderful to be alive and to be able to stand and stare!
>
> (Blaxter 1990: 30)

This woman could be said to have reached what Erikson described as a state of ego integrity and Maslow termed self actualization (Erikson 1965; Maslow 1954), discussed in Chapter 1.

Refined down into broad categories there emerged from the HLS four main explanations for health as well as those who simply could not explain it. (Table 2.3).

Table 2.3 Explanations of health

	Women (%)		Men (%)	
	65–74 years $n = 592$	Over 75 years $n = 344$	65–74 years $n = 448$	Over 75 years $n = 231$
Can't explain	9	14	8	8
Have no disease	10	13	16	16
Have physical energy	14.5	9	12	9
Unable to do things	29	33	26	28
Feel good	57	44	55	51

Source: Health and Lifestyles Survey 1987.

Well over half of the men and women under 75 years expressed their health in terms of feelings, but this was less so for the very old women who were more inclined to think of health in terms of doing things.

In a study of gender differences in health at older ages (Sidell 1991), I used qualitative interview techniques to explore older women's experience of health. It was extremely difficult to categorize their beliefs about and attitudes to health and illness because they would typically express sometimes conflicting beliefs and attitudes at different points in the conversation. However they could 'roughly' be located along a continuum which broadly reflects the explanations identified in the HLS. This continuum goes as follows

Physical–
    functional–
        emotional–
            psychological–
                spiritual.

Rarely were any of their beliefs and attitudes held in exclusion but the women could be located more to one end than the other. Typical of a more physical explanation was this description of health: 'Being free in body to do what you want to do, not to be cramped with rheumatic pains'.

Clearly physical explanations were linked to functional ones with good health described as:

> When you can get about and get your own shopping and not depend on people to run and get your errands and run and do this and you have got to plead with somebody to do something for you.

Yet another woman described her health in terms of moods, it was for her an emotional state: 'Sometimes you would think I am so cheerful, 'cos I'll have a mood and I'll start singing for no reason. I just happen to be'. Others talked of health as feeling confident and some women thought health was a state of mind: 'I don't think you can get rid of cancer by any strength or will power of mind, but I think general health, yes'.

Some held a more spiritual explanation of health, believing that it was a gift from their god. One woman who believed in reincarnation thought that life, health included, was a matter of destiny. It was a process of development which began before, and would go on after, this life. However her concept of destiny was not fatalistic, she believed in a 'law of consequences' – what one did yesterday has consequences for today and the course of development was not fixed: 'I believe that we come with a certain amount of basic ground. There's good ground, and not so good ground, the possibilities to develop'.

The explanations people use especially in later life, to explain health are very likely to be affected by their experience of health and, as Jocelyn Cornwell (1984) points out, to their individual life history. This provides a framework for their understanding of health 'now'. Some aspects of their life history will be shared by others in the same age cohort, the emergence of the welfare state for instance and the experience of two world wars. Others will share experiences which are to do with class, gender or culture. Their explanation of health Cornwell argues is very much bound up with making sense of their individual biographies with all the cross cutting variables of cohort, class, gender and culture.

Anthropological studies of other cultures are rich in accounts of health beliefs and the holistic account of health is highly influenced by eastern cultural beliefs. But there are few studies of the beliefs about health and illness of black and ethnic minority groups in British society throughout the age range. Qureshi (1991) has drawn attention to the influence of religious belief on health beliefs where disease is part of God's will and sometimes punishment. One in-depth study by Jenny Donovan (1986) explored the health beliefs and attitudes of British Asian and Afro-Caribbean people of all ages. Many of her respondents attributed illness to the cold damp climate of Britain which compared unfavourably to the warm, sunny and friendlier atmosphere they associated with their countries of origin.

Rory Williams has worked extensively with older people in Aberdeen over a number of years to explore their attitudes and beliefs about health and illness and to death and dying. Although his methods were qualitative and the interviews like Cornwell's work based on the life history of the individual, his analysis unlike Cornwell's was a cultural one. He was particularly interested in exploring the interactions between religion and culture and patterns of thought. He provides us with a rich source of 'lay logic' (Williams 1983, 1990). Williams is concerned with the 'deeper assumptions underlying health talk'. He identified some very similar basic assumptions made by older Aberdonians about health and illness to those found by Herzlich in Paris and he draws on her work a great deal. He too found three major ways of viewing health:

1 being free from illness or disease;
2 being a source of strength to resist illness; and
3 having the capacity to function in everyday life.

Like Blaxter and Paterson's grandmothers the most significant of these three perspectives for the older Aberdonians was the capacity to function, but health as a strength to resist illness was also very important. This notion of strength and its corollary weakness is a recurring theme amongst lay explanations of health and illness (Cornwell 1984; Wenger 1988). Weakness could be localized to a particular part of the body such as having a 'weak chest' but it was also used in the more metaphorical sense of constitutional vulnerability. As with Blaxter and Paterson's grandmothers there was a strong moral implication to having the strength to resist illness and disease and if not to resisting the disease then at least to not giving in to the symptoms.

Illness behaviour

Much of William's analysis is concerned with how older people in Aberdeen cope with illness or the threat of it. Throughout his analysis Williams reminds us that his respondents rarely operated with unified concepts, that inconsistency was the norm and that 'old people' as exemplified by his sample cannot be seen as one group with common attitudes and beliefs. What Williams does is to identify themes, patterns and dilemmas.

He found five broad premises or assumptions which were held by his respondents in considering how to cope with illness (Williams 1990: 43). These were as follows:

1 Illness as controlled by normal living: 'If I keep up my normal activity, I help myself to prevent or cope with illness', and/or 'If I do not keep up my normal activity, I make my condition worse'.

Carrying on with everyday activities, doing housework, gardening and other essential chores was thought to keep ailments at bay without the need to take on extra physical activity. And this reflects the type of health preventative behaviour found amongst the older respondents to the HLS discussed earlier. The demands of normal living were not only preventative but helped to prevent any condition from deteriorating.

2 Illness as a continuous struggle: 'Even if I am seriously restricted, I do not stop struggling to perform my normal activities'.

'Determination' was the key to overcoming illnesses which were restricting but not serious, such as varicose veins, breathlessness, or back trouble. It was a determination not to give up or lie down to it; this echoes the views of Blaxter and Paterson's grandmothers.

3 Illness as an alternative way of life: 'If I am seriously restricted by illness, I develop alternative interests which offer positive rewards'.

This was not a common response but there were a minority of respondents who, when faced with restrictions which could not be overcome, such as failing eyesight, would listen to 'talking books' or if their mobility was restricted by a stroke they would take up more sedentary activities.

These first three of Williams's categories of response to illness fall very much within the framework of activity theory (Havighurst, 1963) whereas his last two fit more into the framework of disengagement theory (Cumming and Henry, 1961).

4 Illness as a loss to be endured: 'If I am seriously restricted by illness, I am finished', and/or 'If I am seriously restricted by illness, I forget about my past interests', and/or 'If I am seriously restricted by illness, I pass the time with distasteful alternatives'.

This was a much more negative response to illness than the first three, although it was characterized by a sense of stoicism. Being lost or finished refers to the person one once was, who has been wiped out by illness. It was often accompanied by resignation or accepting one's limitations and not hankering after activities one used to do but getting on with things one was still able to do. This acceptance of changed and restricted circumstances helped to prevent resentment and bitterness.

5 Illness as a release from effort: 'If I am restricted by illness, I give some things up with relief'.

There was a degree of ambivalence in this last attitude between self-reproach and deservedness.

As well as these categories Williams noted certain coherent patterns made up from these premises. One which he calls 'illness as exile' was a combination of 1 and 4. This was similar to Herzlich's 'illness as destroyer'. In this type of response illness has to be avoided at all costs because it represents such a threat to the self. A combination of 1 and 2 represented what Williams called 'illness as a test of achievement' and was similar to Herzlich's 'illness as occupation'. Illness either had to be struggled against or struggled with but it was always a preoccupation. Herzlich's category of 'illness as liberator' was also recognizable in Williams's sample and was represented by a combination of 4 and 5 which William's called 'illness as disengagement'. However, Williams is adamant that 'people cannot regularly be typified as exponents of a single coherent pattern of coping' (1990: 49). A strong and consistent theme was the moral connotation of health and illness. This has implications for the question of where responsibility for health lies. Williams identified two dimensions of responsibility. One was the strength to resist illness and the second was the capacity to meet the demands of everyday life. Having constitutional strength was akin to moral fibre and it was mainly one's responsibility to muster this. Many respondents however acknowledged that this had an hereditary component. The capacity or incapacity for tasks was more a mechanical matter imposed by disease and so exempt from responsibility.

The moral aspect of older people's attitudes to health and illness is a common theme. Claire Wenger's study in rural Wales of both working and middle class older people found that: 'Good health is associated with the right attitudes and moral fibre and complaining or talking about health is seen as self-indulgent' (1988: 12,13). Older people's tendency to minimize health problems, Wenger believes, is also in response to ageist attitudes. Older people deny or play down their physical ailments in order not to fulfil negative images and be labelled in stereotypical ways. Williams' thesis on the other hand interprets this tendency to minimize health problems rather differently. He maintains that it is the cultural influence of Calvinist Scotland that accounts for the moral imperative to be in good health. But when Williams explored the concept of old age with his respondents he found that for many 'old' was not a chronological term but was actually synonymous with ill-health. To have ill-health is to be old, therefore to be in good health is to be 'not old' even if one is 70, 80, or even 90. Old age represented failing strength and lowered resistance to disease. 'The blood is thin' 'the body runs down' and loss of energy and 'spirits' were the images associated with 'old': 'the belief that age brought illness was sufficiently entrenched to make it possible, eventually, to make illness the grounds for seeing oneself as 'really' old' (Williams 1990: 63).

This was a strong theme in Thompson et al.'s book (1990) which is actually called *I Don't Feel Old* and based on in-depth interviews with 55 older people. Most of their respondents did not believe that actual age determined if someone was old. Being old was to do with their physical condition – they had internalized the cultural stereotype that old is synonymous with decline and ill-health. Common descriptions of old were:

> When people are incapable of doing what they used to.
>
> It's not what you look like,. There's nothing nicer than an elderly lady with white hair. It's senility, when you lose control of your faculties.
>
> No age when people get old. It's to do with health.
>
> When one becomes unwell.
>
> Depends on health and physical ability.
>
> Well I think old means when you are incapable of doing what you used to do. I think of this one as old because she's a bit helpless at times. But there's another lady more or less as old, but she's capable, so I don't think of her as old.
>
> (Thompson *et al.* 1990: 128)

Denying ill-health is to deny the negative stereotype of old age. Older people are thus under great pressure to cope stoically with ill-health, not to complain and to suffer in silence. They are also under great pressure not to make too many demands upon the health and welfare services and become a burden to the rest of society. Unfortunately attempts to counter ageist attitudes by focusing on those older people who are very fit and healthy such as 90 year old marathon runners inadvertently collude with this pressure on older people to minimize their health problems and to put up with their aches and pains. Rather we need to question the pathogenic paradigm which categorises everyone as either diseased or healthy and to adopt a more salutogenic paradigm in which old age can encompass chronic illness, disability and good health in one person at the same time.

Unfortunately most of the evidence on the health status of old people is firmly rooted in the pathogenic paradigm and the medical model. This abstract statistical evidence is about aggregates and tells us something about everyone but very little about each one. It describes the older population as a whole. What this kind of evidence tells us and how it compares with the available qualitative data is the subject of the next chapter.

3

Patterns of health and illness among older people

Introduction

In Chapter 1 different models of health were identified and these different 'ways of seeing' were related to different 'ways of knowing'. In this chapter we are going to examine the evidence, what we know about the health of the present generation of older people, from objective and subjective accounts. First we will focus on evidence within a biomedical framework and look at objective, hard data on the prevalence of disease before going on to look at subjective accounts of self reported illness and self-assessed health, which give a more social and holistic view. In this chapter we are taking an overview of the health of older people by exploring the evidence on the population of older people and groups within it. In Part 2 we will examine individual experiences of health and illness.

The medical model of health relies mainly on statistical data on mortality and morbidity to take stock of the health of the population. National statistics on death and the diseases which caused deaths are collected annually and provide information on trends and changes in the patterns of death and disease. From this type of evidence we can discern the death and disease profiles of the population of older people in aggregate, and we can make comparisons between certain groups of older people on the basis of gender, class and sometimes ethnicity.

The death profile of older people

Paradoxically mortality, i.e. death, statistics are the most widely used source of evidence on the health status of the general population. Since death registration began in 1841 information on the mortality of the population has

Table 3.1 Standardized mortality ratios of males in Great Britain

	15–64	65–74	75+
Class I	66	68	73
Class II	77	81	84
Class IIIn	105	86	92
Class IIIm	96	100	105
Class IV	109	106	108
Class V	124	109	116
Ratio-Class V/Class I	1.88	1.60	1.59

Source: Fox *et al.* (1985) Table 2, cited in Victor (1993)

Table 3.2 Summary of main findings on immigrant mortality study in England and Wales, 1970–78

Mortality by cause	*Comparison with death rates for England and Wales*
Tuberculosis	*high* in immigrants from India subcontinent, Ireland, Caribbean, Africa and Scotland.
Liver cancer	*high* in immigrants from India subcontinent, Caribbean and Africa.
Cancer of stomach, large intestine, breast	*low* mortality among Indians.
Ischaemic heart disease	*high* mortality found in immigrants from Indian subcontinent.
Hypertension and stroke	*strikingly high* mortality among immigrants from the Caribbean and Africa – 4 to 6 times higher for hypertension and twice as high for strokes as the level in England and Wales.
Diabetes	*high* among immigrants born in the Caribbean and Indian subcontinent.
Obstructive lung disease (including chronic bronchitis)	*low* in all immigrants in comparison to ratio for England and Wales.
Maternal mortality	*high* in immigrants from Africa, Caribbean, and to a lesser extent the Indian subcontinent.
Violence and accidents	*high* in all immigrant groups.

Source: Whitehead 1987 taken from Marmot *et al.* (1984).

been provided by the death certificate. This records the name, sex, age, date and place of death, place of birth, final occupation and marital status. It also records the main cause of death as defined by a qualified medical practitioner using the international classification of diseases (ICD). The Office of Population

Censuses and Surveys OPCS analyse and publish these data annually. From these data we can discover gender and class differences in death rates and the causes of death of older men and women.

The majority of deaths in western societies take place in old age and this is considered a distinct health gain and a mark of socioeconomic progress. In fact death has become largely the concern of older people in this society in the last half of this century. Before the twentieth century it was commonplace for a child to experience the death of a sibling either in infancy or childhood and women faced the high probability that they would die in childbirth. Now deaths in infancy are rare, even rarer is death in childbirth. Until the spread of AIDS we have not been at the mercy of epidemics and although life threatening diseases have not been eliminated, most people can reasonably expect to live out their 'span'. Death is put off until old age, we rarely encounter it and we do not have to think about it. As 79 per cent of all deaths in Britain in 1987 were of people over the age of 65 mortality data largely tells us about older people.

Mortality statistics have provided much of the evidence on inequalities in health mainly based on social class (Townsend and Davidson 1986; Whitehead 1987). Whilst acknowledging that establishing the social class of older people and particularly older women is extremely difficult (Estes *et al.* 1984; Arber and Ginn 1991a, 1993), all the available evidence suggests that the class differentials in mortality persist into later life as Table 3.1 shows. (It uses the Registrar General's classification on occupation. Class I includes professional occupations, Class II, service and managerial occupations, Class IIIn, skilled manual occupations, Class IV, semi-skilled manual occupations and Class V unskilled occupations.)

Data on mortality for black and minority ethnic older people is even harder to locate mainly because proportionately they have not formed a large enough group to be statistically visible in national survey data.

A major study of immigrant mortality in England and Wales was carried out by Marmot *et al.* (1984). There is a tendency for people who migrate to be 'healthier' than those who stay behind and recent immigrants have lower mortality rates than the host population. This was the case in Marmot's study except for immigrants from Ireland who had higher mortality rates than people in Ireland and in England and Wales. A summary of the main findings from the Marmot study was presented by Whitehead (1987) and is reprinted in Table 3.2.

One of the most striking features of the death profile of older people is the gender imbalance. As Figure 3.1 shows women outlive men in Britain throughout the older age range and have done so since records began in 1841. This is also the case for every country which keeps records as Figure 3.2 shows.

In no country is the male/female difference reversed. There is on average a difference in life-expectancy of about six to seven years at birth and three years at age 65. In some countries this is narrower, such as Greece and Cuba, yet in others such as France the gap is wider with women outliving men by just over eight years. The reasons why there is this national variation is beyond the scope of this book but women's greater longevity in general has been the subject of much debate.

The precise reasons for women's greater longevity remains unclear but several reasons have been suggested (Waldron 1976, 1982; Verbrugge 1983; Gove 1973). These include:

36 *The health context*

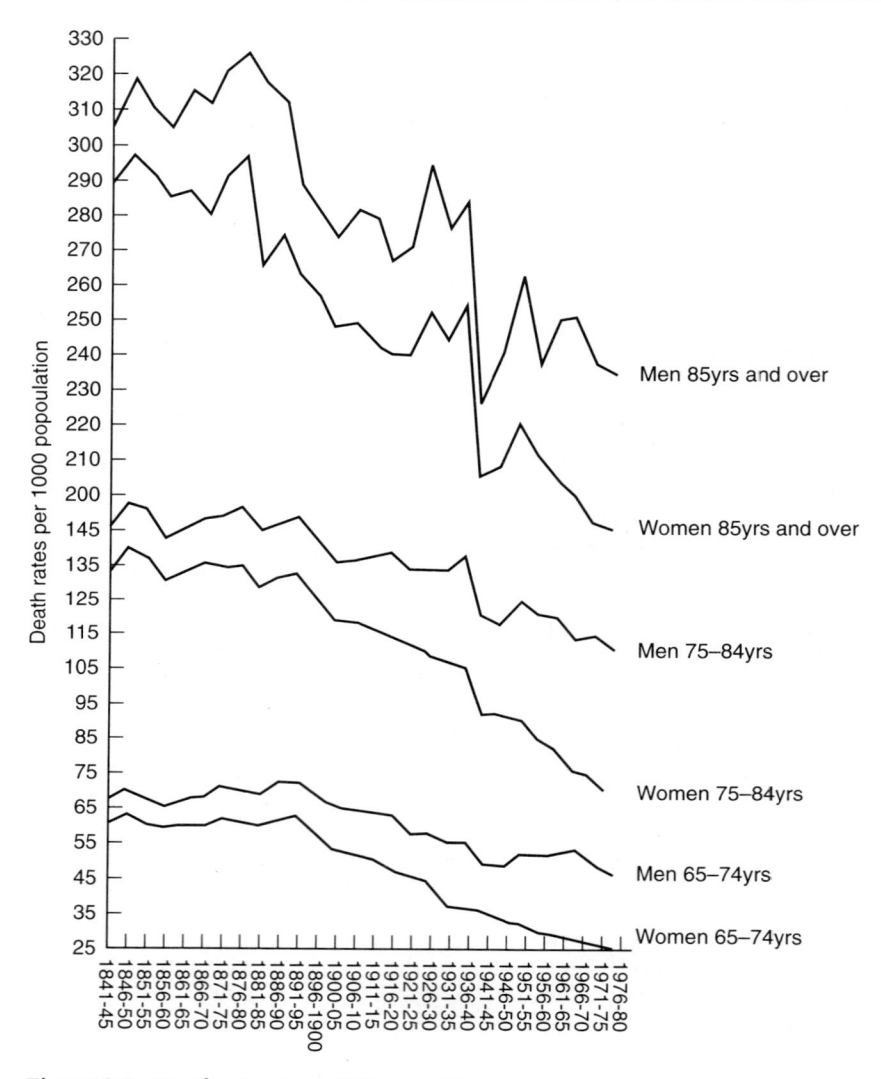

Figure 3.1 Death rates since 1841 over 65 years.
Source: OPCS 1989

- sex linked physical differences;
- different responses to environmental hazards;
- different health habits, for example smoking and drinking;
- personality differences – men are said to be more aggressive and willing to take risks;
- differences in reactions to illness and disability, therefore conditions are diagnosed earlier in women.

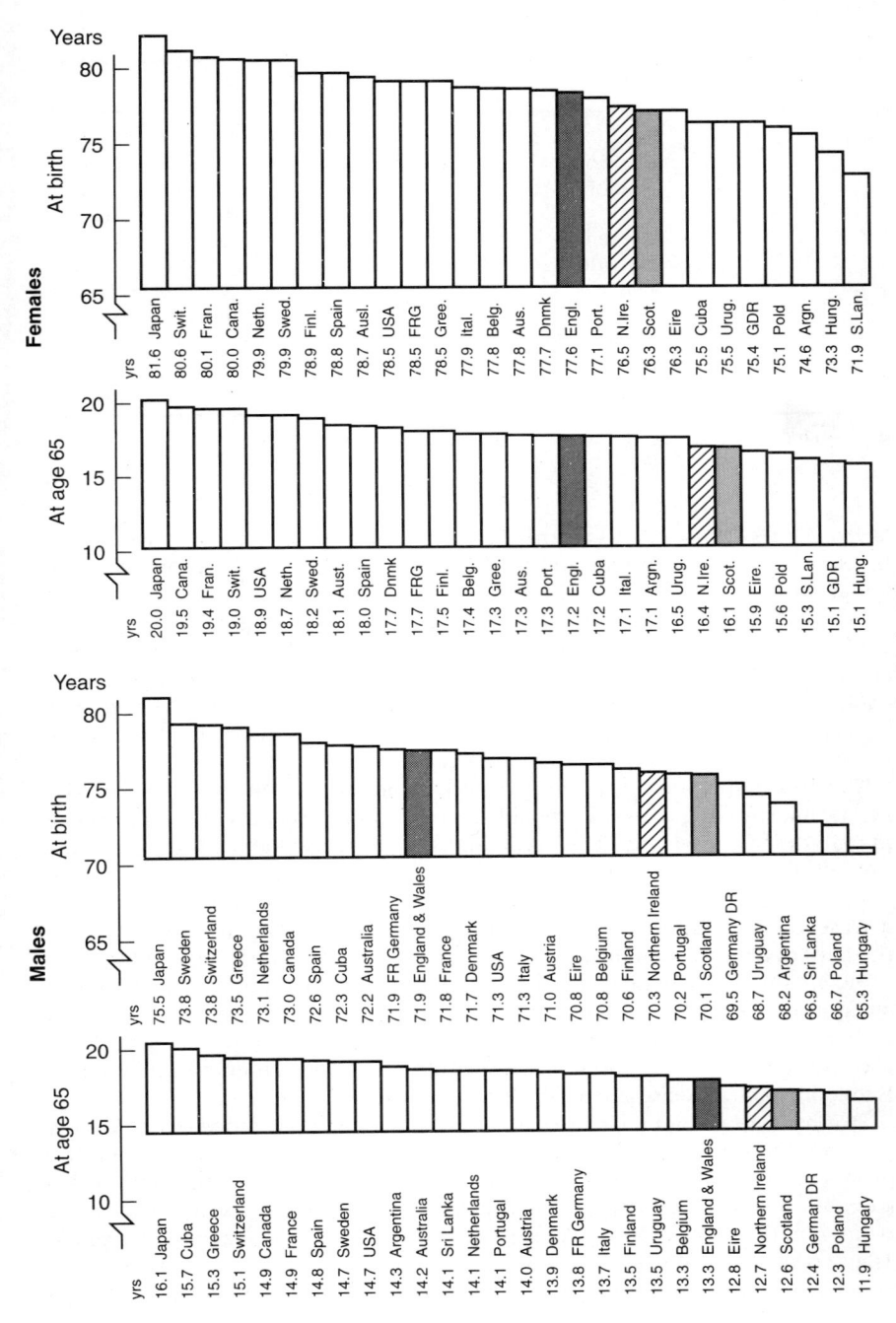

Figure 3.2 Life expectancy in selected countries at age 65 and at birth, 1985.
Source: WHO, *World Health Statistics 1987*, WHO Geneva, 1987.

38   The health context

Table 3.3 Death rate per thousand population for men and women over 55, by age group, England and Wales, 1971–89

		55–64	65–74	75–84	85+
1971	Men	20.1	50.5	113.0	231.8
	Women	10.0	26.1	73.6	185.7
	Sex ratio (M/F)	2.01	1.93	1.54	1.25
1981	Men	17.7	45.6	105.2	226.5
	Women	9.5	24.1	66.2	178.2
	Sex ratio (M/F)	1.86	1.89	1.59	1.27
1989	Men	14.8	39.5	95.7	195.7
	Women	8.8	22.6	60.3	162.4
	Sex ratio (M/F)	1.68	1.75	1.59	1.21
% decrease 1971–89	Men	26.4	21.8	15.37	15.6
	Women	12.0	13.4	18.1	12.5

Source: OPCS (1990), Table 13, cited in Arber and Ginn (1991c)

Myrna Lewis (1985: 6,7) assessing the evidence claims that 'the overwhelming factors appear to be smoking and alcohol', but that 'the greater durability of the female body remains a piece of the answer'.

Women's mortality advantage over men is greatest among the 'young old' as Table 3.3 shows. The mortality rate for men between the ages of 55 and 74 is about twice that of women in 1971 and about 70 per cent higher in 1989. But Table 3.3 also shows that the decline in mortality over the last 20 years has been greater for men than for women and could well be related to the decline in smoking amongst men.

The information on causes of death adds weight to the conclusion reached by Lewis that smoking patterns probably account for a good deal of the difference in male/female longevity. This is corroborated by the evidence showing that a preponderance of male deaths are concentrated in the heart–lung system. However men and women die basically from the same main four causes; heart disease, cancer, respiratory disease and cerebro-vascular disease or strokes. It is the pace of death which differs rather than the reasons (Verbrugge 1989).

Fig 3.3 shows the main causes of death for men and women broken down by age groups. Heart disease is the main cause of death for both men and women over the age of 65 and this is consistent through the upper age groups, it accounts consistently for about a third of the deaths of all men and all women. Ischaemic heart disease accounts for most of these deaths.

Deaths from malignancies are the next cause of death for men over 65 years but only the third overall cause of death for women over 65. For women the proportions of deaths from cancer diminish in the older age groups. This is also true, but to a lesser extent, for men. The percentage of deaths from cancer for women in the three older age groups drops from 31 per cent at 65–74 years to 18 per cent at 75–84 years and down to 10 per cent of womens' deaths over 85 years. For men the percentages are 29 to 23 to 14 per cent respectively. Within the malignancy group, cancer of the respiratory tract affects proportionately

Major causes of death Men

(Graph showing % of all male deaths by age group 65–74yrs, 75–84yrs, Over 85yrs)
- Heart disease
- Malignant neoplasms
- Respiratory disease
- Cerebrovascular disease
- Circulatory disease

65–74yrs n = 44298
75–84yrs n = 104053
Over 85yrs n = 223133

Major causes of death Women

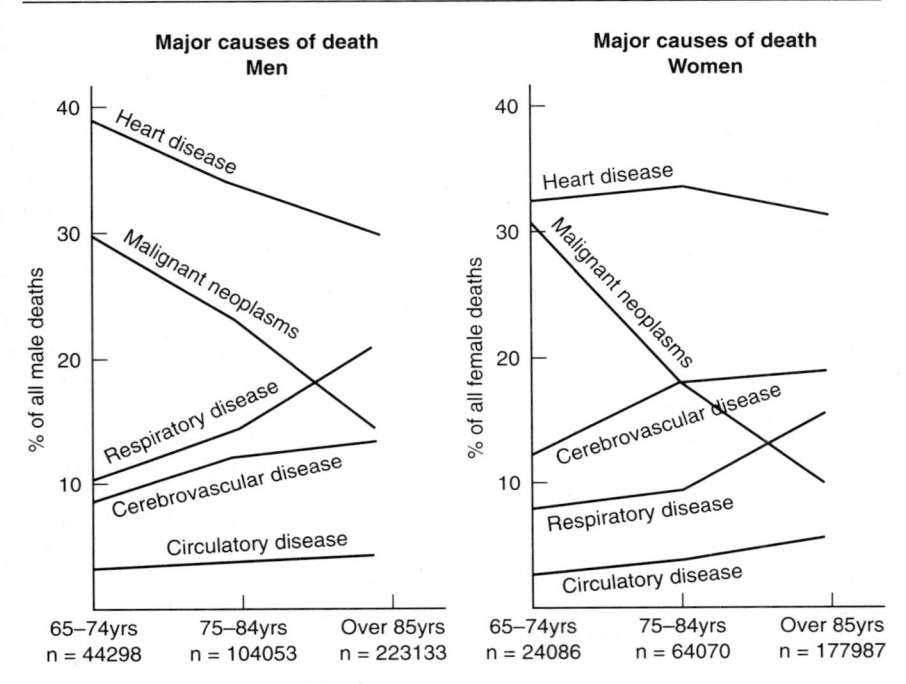

(Graph showing % of all female deaths by age group 65–74yrs, 75–84yrs, Over 85yrs)
- Heart disease
- Malignant neoplasms
- Cerebrovascular disease
- Respiratory disease
- Circulatory disease

65–74yrs n = 24086
75–84yrs n = 64070
Over 85yrs n = 177987

Figure 3.3 Major causes of death.
Source: National Mortality Statistics, OPCS, 1989.

more men than women in all the older age groups. The other significant group of malignancies that is notably different for men and women is that of the genitourinary tract. This is the cause of a greater proportion of male deaths than female deaths, especially at the two older age groups. It is very much a reversal of the patterns of younger age groups. Although some of the difference can be accounted for by the larger number of male deaths from cancer of the bladder, much of the difference is due to cancer of the prostate, which is almost non existent before the age of 65 years, but causes an increasingly high proportion of male deaths over the age of 75 years. On the other hand deaths from cancer of specifically female organs are relatively high from the age of 25 onwards but proportionately diminish in old age.

Whilst cancer is the second largest cause of death for men over the age of 65 years, for women death from cerebrovascular disease is the second largest cause and this proportionately increases with age. Cerebrovascular disease in all its forms, subarachnoid haemorrhage, intra-cerebral and intra-cranial haemorrhage, cerebral infarction, cerebral atherosclerosis and acute cerebrovascular disease account for a higher proportion of all female deaths over 65 than male deaths and this difference increases at the older age groups.

Non-malignant respiratory disease is the third highest cause of male deaths and the fourth highest cause of female deaths. But within the range of respiratory diseases there are marked male and female differences.

Proportionately more women than men die from acute respiratory disease, particularly pneumonia, which could well be masking other conditions. In contrast proportionately more men die from chronic respiratory diseases. This, combined with the larger number of male deaths from cancer of the respiratory tract, again points to the influence of smoking on that generation of older men.

Deaths from circulatory diseases show very similar patterns for both men and women, being the fifth largest cause of death for men and women at all the older age groups. Within the category of circulatory diseases, atherosclerosis is an important cause of death for women over 85 years.

Other than these five main causes of death there are an increasing number of deaths in the older age groups for both men and women recorded under 'mental illness'. Whilst most of these deaths are attributed to senile organic psychosis, there remain a small number of older people, and particularly very old women who die, according to the records, of 'other psychosis', 'neurotic disorders', 'personality disorder' and other non psychotic mental disorders which include acute reaction to stress and adjustment reaction as well as depression. It is difficult to see how people actually die from these conditions and in some cases the terms are probably used euphemistically for suicide. But it confirms popular mythology, that people can 'lose the will to live' or die of a 'broken heart'.

Of the remaining disease systems the digestive, the nervous, the musculo-skeletal and the endocrine, metabolic, nutritional and immunity disorders all cause proportionately more deaths amongst older women than older men. In fact, although heart disease is the major cause of death for women as well as men, a higher proportion of women's deaths are spread throughout the disease categories. And many of the diseases from which a higher proportion of women than men die are those diseases which are likely to be more symptomatic prior to death, for example cerebrovascular disease, atherosclerosis, dementia and diseases of the musculo-skeletal system. Clearly this has implications for the health care of older women and this aspect will be addressed in Part 3 of this book. The highly symptomatic nature of older women's health problems becomes even clearer when we look at the morbidity statistics.

Morbidity

If people are living longer, are they also healthier in medical terms, i.e. are they without disease and illness? This was the second component of Fries's thesis, discussed in the Introduction, that morbidity is compressed into a very short time at the end of a long life, that most people are living to the age of 80 or 90 free from illness or disability until they suffer from the illness from which they will die in a fairly short time. The arguments for or against Fries's compression of morbidity thesis are inconclusive (Bebbinton 1988; Rogers *et al.* 1990) and have been reviewed in Arber and Ginn (1991c). They used data from the General Household Survey (GHS) to compare disability rates amongst older people over time, between 1980 and 1985. They found that there was a fall of about 10 per cent in the proportions of men in their 80s who were severely

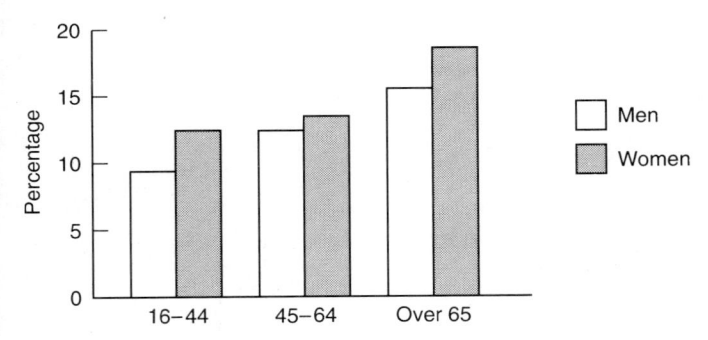

Figure 3.4 Acute sickness in population of Great Britain, 1991.
Source: General Household Survey, OPCS, 1993.

disabled but no change in the proportions of women. In fact all the evidence suggests that women pay a price for their increased longevity in terms of increased levels of non-life-threatening but highly symptomatic diseases such as arthritis (Verbrugge 1984, 1989). Verbrugge has argued that medical technology has increased the life span of people with previously life threatening conditions but 'ill people have been saved, rather than well people being rewarded by disease absence across their life span' (Verbrugge 1989: 29).

Acute health problems

Acute health problems, unlike chronic conditions, are of short-term duration or at least they are problems which are resolvable. Infections and colds and flu come into this category. The prevalence of acute health problems does increase with age as Figure 3.4 indicates.

However included in this category are broken bones and all accidents, injury and poisoning. The incidence of these show a disturbing rise amongst the older population especially older women. Figures 3.5 and 3.6 show the numbers hospitalized for injury and poisoning and the consultation rates to GPs.

Young men and older women have the highest rates of injury and poisoning. Much of this, for older women, is accounted for by fractures which may be attributed to osteoporosis (Smith 1992) although not entirely so. Older people are prone to falling and this has been linked to a range of factors, such as hypothermia or the over prescribing of tranquillizers or drugs for hypertension which can make people dizzy. In fact older people suffer a great deal of toxic effects from prescribed drugs (Burns and Phillipson 1986) which may be correctly or incorrectly administered. Much of this injury and poisoning then is iatrogenically induced.

Chronic illness and disability

A chronic illness, unlike an acute illness, is of long duration and there is no effective cure. Evidence in Britain on the incidence of chronic illness and

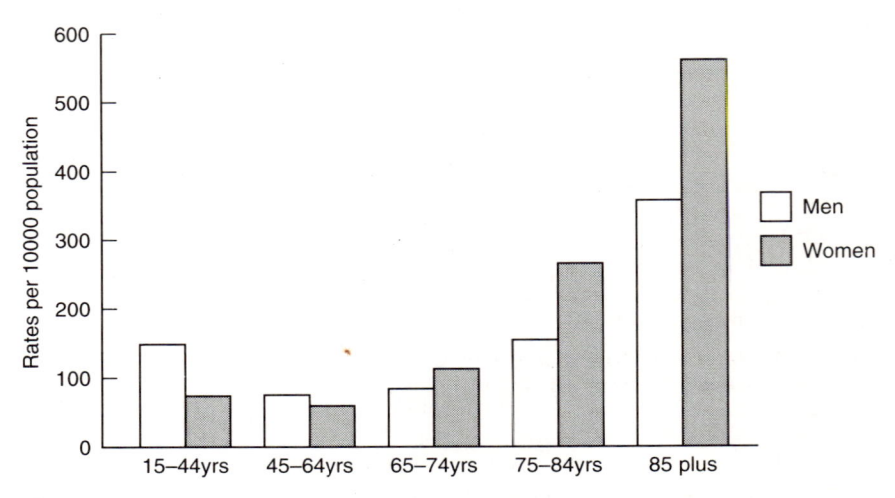

Figure 3.5 Accidents, injury and poisoning: All discharges and deaths.
Source: OPCS, 1987.

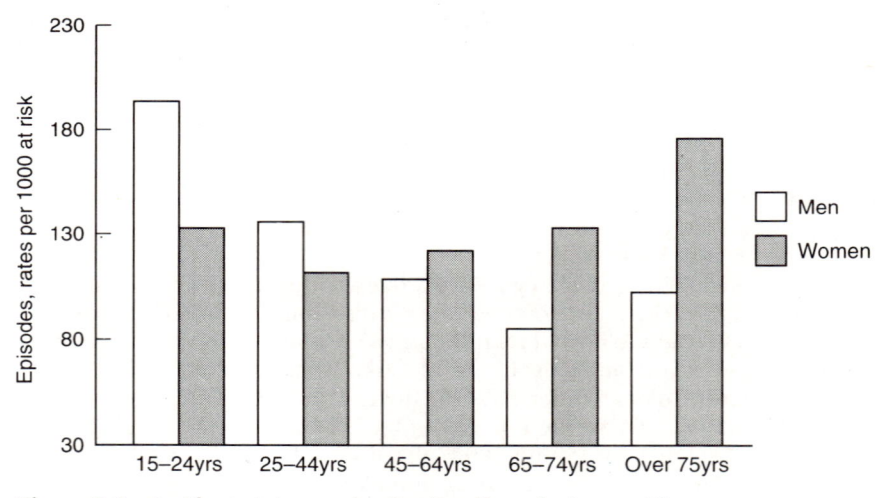

Figure 3.6 Accidents, injury and poisoning: Consultations to GPs.
Source: Royal College of General Practitioners, 1986.

disability is collected annually by the GHS and published by OPCS. This is a nationally representative sample survey of around 14,000 people which includes about 4,000 people over the age of 65. Respondents are asked first if they have a long standing illness or disability. Those who respond in the affirmative are asked if it limits their normal activities. Thus the GHS makes an important distinction between having a chronic illness and experiencing disability. Analysis of the GHS data for 1990 shows how the prevalence of a

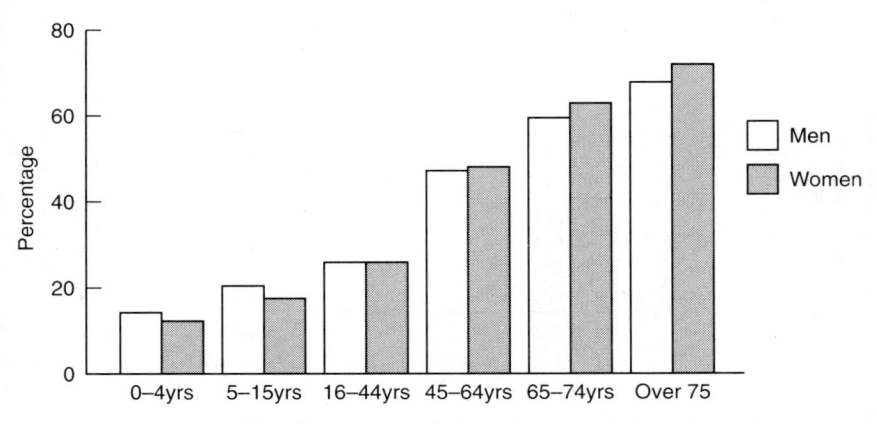

Figure 3.7 Long standing illness in population of Great Britain, 1990. *Source:* OPCS, 1993.

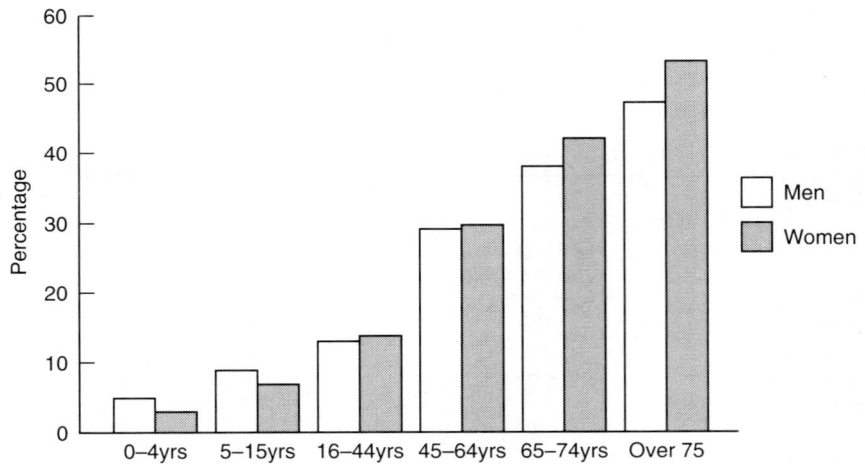

Figure 3.8 Limiting long standing illness in population of Great Britain, 1990. *Source:* OPCS, 1993.

long standing illness increases with age as well as the incidence of a long standing limiting illness (see Figures 3.7 and 3.8).

Data from the OPCS disability survey (Martin *et al.* 1988) which consisted of four separate surveys carried out between 1985 and 1988 shows an even greater prevalence of chronic illness and disability. This survey interviewed people both in the community and in institutions, unlike the GHS which is a community only survey. Variations in methodology and the absence of institutionalized older people from the GHS would account for the smaller proportions suffering from a chronic illness. This evidence is compared in Figure 3.9.

44 The health context

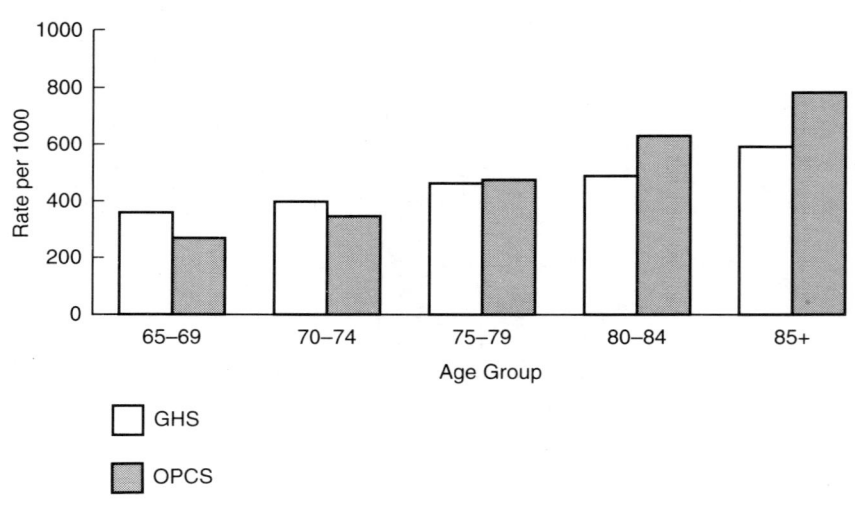

Figure 3.9 Disability and chronic illness prevalence by age in population aged 65+, 1988
Source: Martin et al, 1988.

Table 3.4 Reported long standing illness

Percentage reporting	Women 65–74 n = 592	Women 75 and over n = 344	Men 65–74 n = 448	Men 75 and over n = 231
Arthritis	17.5	20.0	8.0	7.0
Heart disease	9.5	12.0	12.0	11.0
High blood pressure	8.5	10.5	7.5	7.0
Orthopaedic condition	3.5	4.0	2.5	5.0
Back trouble	4.0	4.0	3.0	1.5
Sight	3.0	4.0	4.0	3.5
Stroke	2.5	3.5	4.0	4.0
Bronchitis	3.0	3.0	5.0	7.0
Diabetes	3.0	2.0	.5	3.0
Gastric/intestinal	2.0	2.0	2.0	1.0
Depression	2.0	1.5	0.2	—
Thyroid	1.5	1.5	0.2	—
Respiratory disease	1.5	2.0	2.5	3.5
Deafness	1.0	2.5	2.5	3.5
Cancer	1.5	1.5	1.0	1.0
Hernia	1.5	1.5	1.0	2.5
Stomach ulcer	1.5	1.0	2.5	2.0
Anaemia	1.0	1.5	1.5	1.5
Genito-urinal	0.5	2.0	1.0	3.0

Source: Health and Lifestyles Survey 1987; own analysis of unpublished data

What are the illnesses being reported? The GHS does not break down their overall category of chronic illnesses by specific illnesses but the Health and Lifestyles Survey (HLS) does. Table 3.4 shows the actual illness reported by men and women broken down by age groups.

There are some marked male/female differences. Many more women than men have arthritis. But also the percentage of women reporting arthritis rises with age whereas for men it decreases. In fact this tendency for women's illnesses to increase with age and for men's to decrease reflects a general trend in all the illnesses. There are some exceptions. For women, diabetes, depression and stomach ulcers diminish with age. For men, orthopaedic conditions, diabetes, respiratory diseases, deafness, hernias and diseases of the genito-urinary systems increase with age. This indicates that men who survive into old age do not, like the women, tend to accumulate highly symptomatic diseases and conditions.

As we noted earlier large national sample surveys do not include a large enough percentage of older people from ethnic minority communities to allow for a separate analysis of health status. As Blakemore and Boneham comment:

> so while evidence is accumulating, either from local community health or social surveys, it is the lack of a full national picture that is startling.
> (Blakemore and Boneham 1993: 94)

Blakemore and Boneham review the evidence that we have from these local surveys and warn against treating older black and minority ethnic older people 'as exotic specimens of ageing among whom there are completely distinctive patterns of health and disease' (ibid.: 160). Drawing on a range of studies (Bhalla and Blakemore 1981; Blakemore 1982; Ebrahim *et al.* 1987 and Cruickshank *et al.* 1980) they piece together the information on the health status of black and minority ethnic older people. Older Afro-Caribbeans experience a higher incidence of strokes compared to whites born in Britain but a lower incidence of heart attacks. Older Asian people are more likely to suffer heart attacks than strokes. A higher than average rate of diabetes has been identified amongst the Afro-Caribbean and Asian populations. Osteoporosis or brittle bone disease which frequently results in fractures in old people, especially women, is more prevalent amongst older whites and Asians than Afro-Caribbeans. Older Asians have an above average risk of contracting or developing tuberculosis and there are relatively high rates of sight problems especially but not entirely due to cataracts amongst older Asian and Afro-Caribbean people. Dental problems and problems with feet and mobility were all noted. Blakemore and Bonham discuss the complexities of assessing the evidence but overall they conclude that although the population of black older people is on the whole younger than the white population, 'the health of older black people is not as good as might be expected' and it is 'no better than that among older white pensioners'. When trying to find explanations and causes why this should be so they thoroughly endorse Alison Norman's (1985) assertion that older black and minority ethnic people's health and well-being is seriously affected by the 'triple jeopardy' of age discrimination, socioeconomic disadvantage, and discrimination in access to services because of language and culture.

Table 3.5 Older respondents with a long standing illness or disability

	Women over 65 n = 2090 % Yes	Limits Activity	Men over 65 n = 1436 % Yes	Limits Activity
All	60	73	56	71
Age groups				
65–74 years	56	68	55	70
75–84 years	64	76	57	73
Over 85 years	71	86	63	82
Marital status				
Married	55	72	56	69
Single	57	72	52	86
Widowed	64	74	59	73
Social class				
Non-manual	57	70	49	64
Manual	63	76	59	76
Housing classes				
Rents from local authority	64	76	60	76
Owner occupier	55	69	53	66
Other rental	61	71	59	76
Education				
Some qualifications	44	58	52	65
No qualifications	57	66	58	73
Self assessed health				
Good	31	45	33	44
Fairly good	66	68	64	71
Not good	92	90	90	91

Source: GHS 1985; own analysis of unpublished data

A more social model of health is concerned with the relationship between the level of chronic illness and disability and socioeconomic variables. Although the GHS has not attempted ethnic monitoring of its sample, it does allow for some secondary analysis of other variables. This enables researchers to discover the relationship of a limited number of other socioeconomic variables such as marital status, social class, housing tenure as well as education, although the question on educational levels is not asked of people over the age of 69 and so it is of limited use. This analysis indicates that the experience of chronic illness and disability in old age differs according to all of these variables. Widowed people experience more chronic illness and disability of a limiting kind than married or single people. Those from non-manual occupational backgrounds experience less than those in manual occupations and those living in local authority rented accommodation experience more than those who own their own houses. Similarly those who lack formal

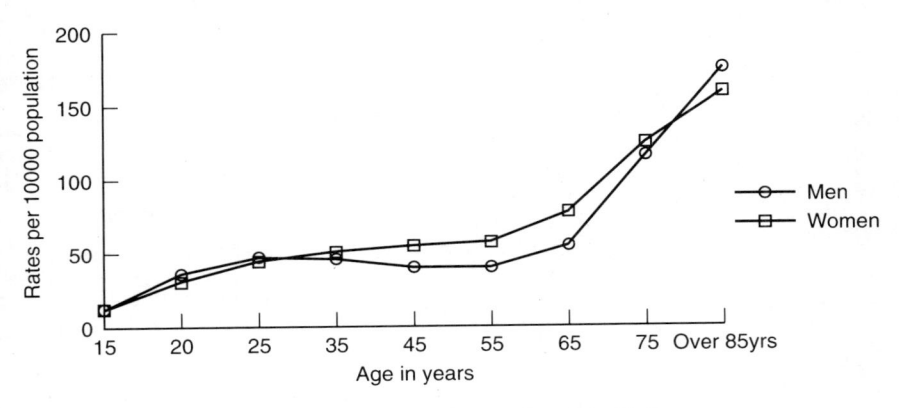

Figure 3.10 Admissions to mental illness hospitals 1986: All diagnoses.
Source: DHSS, 1987. Mental Illness Statistics, England.

educational qualifications suffer more than those who had such qualifications. The picture is a familiar one confirming that social disadvantage continues to affect health status into old age (Taylor and Ford 1983; Arber and Ginn 1991a). Indeed it would be surprising if it did not. It is important, however, to remind ourselves constantly of the diversity of experience within the older population in order to break down both overly negative and overly positive myths and stereotypes of older people in terms of their health. The picture is very different for a working class widow living in local authority accommodation who left school at the minimum age with no formal qualifications than it is for a middle class university educated, married woman of around 65 years living in her own house. Similar distinctions can be made within the older male population. A social model of health is less likely to lead to the attribution of chronic illness and disability to age and more likely to focus on the role of economic and social disadvantage determining health chances and to the impact of loneliness and isolation. This is frequently the experience of older widows.

The incidence of mental illness in older people

The GHS does not differentiate between physical and mental illness but there is evidence that older people suffer more mental illness than younger people and this is reflected in the figures on admission to mental illness hospitals. The graph in Figure 3.10 shows this clearly.

The pie charts in Figure 3.11 give the diagnosis for which older people were admitted to mental illness hospitals. Whilst the actual numbers of women admitted overall is greater than men, 12,234 women to 6,935 men, this only reflects the greater numbers of older women in the population and we need to remember that these admissions represent only a minority of all older people. What the charts show is that men and women suffer from specific mental conditions in roughly the same proportions. There is not a specifically male or female mental condition. Dementia is the largest category for both men and

48 The health context

Women over 65yrs
- 3807 (31%)
- 971 (8%)
- 1368 (11%)
- 237 (2%)
- 600 (5%)
- 1933 (16%)
- 708 (6%)
- 2610 (21%)

Men over 65yrs
- 2154 (31%)
- 438 (6%)
- 1015 (15%)
- 163 (2%)
- 214 (3%)
- 979 (14%)
- 276 (4%)
- 1696 (24%)

- ☐ Affective psychosis
- ▓ Senile dementia
- ░ Other psychosis
- ▧ Neurotic disorders
- ☺ Depressive disorders
- ≡ Schizophrenia
- ■ Personality disorders
- ▨ Other mental illness

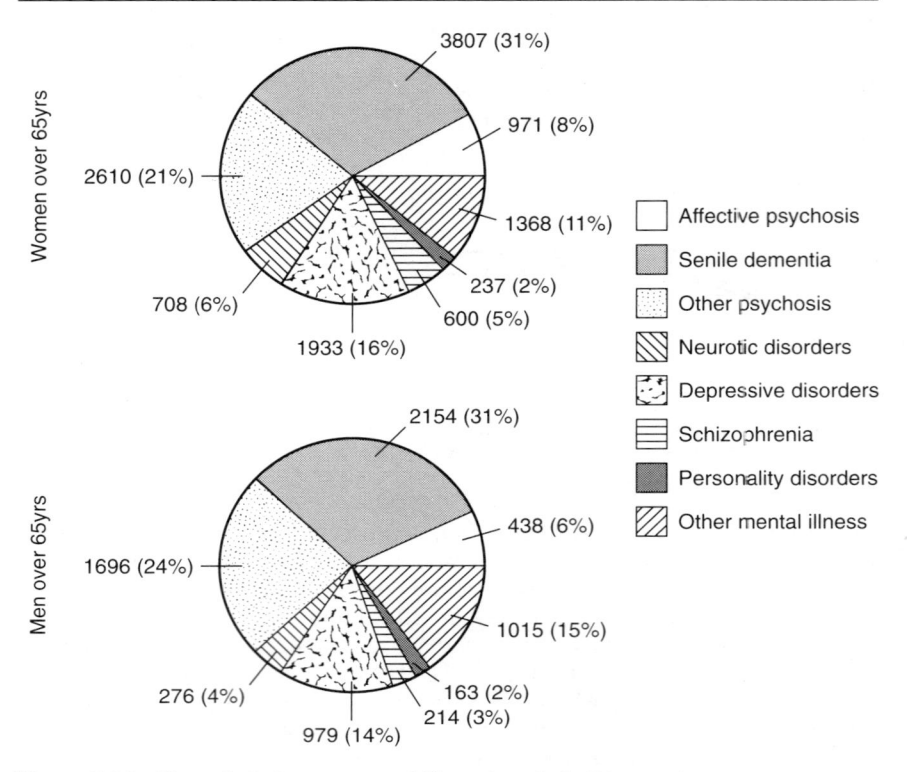

Figure 3.11 First admissions to mental illness hospitals: Diagnostic group.
Source: DHSS, 1989. Mental Illness Statistics, England.

women with 'other psychosis' being the second largest category again for men and women. This somewhat ragbag category includes: paranoid and other hallucinatory states induced by drugs, pathological states induced by drugs and some rather vague categories listed as depressive type, excitative type, reactive confusion, acute paranoid reaction and psychogenic paranoid psychosis. It seems that large numbers of older people are being admitted to hospital with a very unsatisfactory diagnosis. The third largest category of admission is for depression with a slightly higher proportion of women in this category. Affective psychosis is the fourth highest category for both men and women and is made up almost entirely of manic depressive psychosis. Neurotic disorders are slightly higher for women and so is schizophrenia. Surprisingly personality and behavioural disorders normally thought to be more prevalent amongst men are much the same for men and women. It is possible that some of these are undiagnosed dementia.

It is interesting that older men and women are admitted to hospital with a mental illness in much the same proportions when proportionately many more women at all ages consult their GP with mental conditions. The graph in Figure 3.12 shows the consultation rates for mental illness to GPs and the gap between men's and women's consultations is maintained into old age.

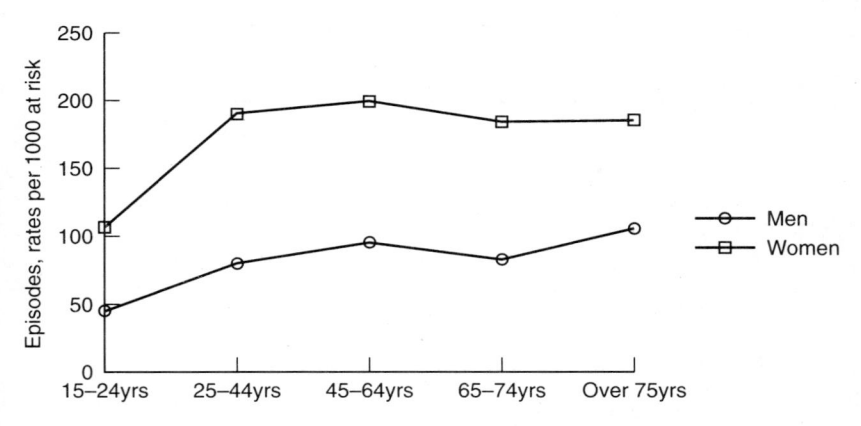

Figure 3.12 Mental disorders: Consultations to GPs.
Source: Royal College of General Practitioners, 1986.

What is clear is that women of all ages visit their GPs with a good deal of symptomatology of a psychological nature. There is a clear discrepancy, however, which is consistent for all the categories of mental illness, that whilst many more women are diagnosed as suffering from mental illness than men, more men are hospitalized. What are the implications of this? Are men or women being discriminated against? The answer to that question depends on whether hospitalization for a mental condition is considered advantageous or disadvantageous. In the case of the black population it is argued that their proportionately greater incarceration for mental illness is a result of racism and racial stereotypes (Pilgrim and Rogers 1993). If we look at the issue from a medical perspective a hospital bed represents a scarce resource and it is doctors who are allocating that resource. Are they doing so unfairly in terms of gender? Are women's conditions not taken as seriously as men's? Are they in fact not as 'real'? There are two separate issues. One is about whether the predominantly male medical profession is more willing to label women as mentally ill, but consider women's mental illness to be less serious than men's as Helen Roberts suggests (1985). The other issue is concerned with what we mean by 'real' illness. How far are GPs, working within a biomedical tradition, constrained by the need to diagnose and treat, and how far then are the diagnoses convenient labels for social, psychological or emotional distress? A more social and holistic model of health would lead to a different understanding of these symptoms of mental malaise and look to different causal relationships. What are the subjective symptoms that are reported by older women and how do they differ from the subjective symptoms of older men?

Subjective experience of health and illness

Self-reported symptoms

Prevalence rates for medically diagnosed diseases do not necessarily tell us anything about the subjective experience of sickness or health. The two do not

Table 3.6 Prevalence reported during the past month of selected mental symptoms in the population over 65 in Great Britain

	Women All % n = 936	Men All % n = 697
Difficulty sleeping	41	23
Worry	28	11
Always tired	26	17
Difficulty concentrating	17	11
Suffers from nerves	17	6
Feels lonely	14	10
Feels bored	13	11
Feels under strain	6	4

Source: Health and Lifestyles Survey 1987; own analysis of unpublished data

Table 3.7 Prevalence reported during the past month of selected physical symptoms in the population over 65 in Great Britain

% Reporting	Women n = 936	Men n = 697
Painful joints	45	30
Eye trouble	31	18
Bad back	29	18
Palpitations	29	24
Foot trouble	28	18
Flu/colds	26	26
Headaches	24	13
Stomach trouble	23	19
Ear trouble	19	21
Sinus trouble	17	16
Constipation	16	11
Faints	14	8
Cough	11	14
Kidney/bladder trouble	8	8

Source: Health and Lifestyles Survey 1987; own analysis of unpublished data

necessarily correspond. It is possible to experience symptoms which are not translated into medically diagnosed disease and not all diagnosed disease is symptomatic.

The Health and Lifestyles Survey (HLS) attempted to identify the symptoms experienced by their respondents in the month previous to the survey interview. Tables 3.6 gives the prevalence of mental symptoms.

Older women report more symptoms of mental malaise than men. Many of these symptoms such as difficulty in sleeping, loneliness or difficulty in concentrating could in some cases be due to bereavement. Worry and feeling under stress could be due to financial hardship or worry over failing physical health. Elaine Murphy (1982) identified chronic physical symptoms such as pain or immobility as a major factor in the incidence of depression in older people, and older women report more physical symptoms than men as Table 3.7 shows.

Older women report more symptoms of a somatic and psychic kind than older men. Biology and physiology represent part of the difference, but much of the difference can be explained with reference to the social environment and women's roles throughout the life-course (Lewis 1985). Two broad explanations of this have been suggested. One is that women's roles are 'more compatible' with getting sick (Nathanson 1975), they have fewer role obligations that cannot be changed (Marcus and Seeman 1981) and they are more willing to report symptoms than men because they are given cultural permission to do so (Phillips and Segal 1969). The implication is that women's illnesses are not 'real' and the difference is just one of willingness to report and opportunity to take on the sick role. The other explanation is based on the assumption that women's illnesses are 'real' and that they are related to women's nurturant roles which are so demanding that the attendant stresses result in more women than men suffering from these highly symptomatic but less serious conditions in the life-threatening sense (Gove and Hughes 1979). There are problems with these explanations; they do not differentiate between women on the basis of marital status, class, age, employment status, sexual orientation, or ethnic origin. Lewis maintains that 'the jury is still out' and Christina Victor (1991:74) notes that, 'It seems likely that several factors account for the gender differences in morbidity and that there are different explanations for different types of illness'. However, in spite of reporting a high level of symptomatology older women are nevertheless optimistic about their general health when asked to give an account of this.

Self-assessed health

The evidence available to assess how older people rate their own health comes from two sources. One is from sample surveys such as the GHS and the HLS. The other is from small scale qualitative studies mostly based on face to face, in-depth and biographical interviews some, but not all, focusing specifically on health issues (Cornwell and Gearing 1989; Thompson *et al.* 1990; Sidell 1991; Bury and Holmes 1991).

Sample surveys ask people some variation of the standard question 'how do you rate your health?'. Their rating is fitted into a three or four point scale ranging from very good to very poor. Inevitably this is a crude measurement but it does provide a generalized picture. The assessments made of their own health by the older respondents to the HLS and the GHS are shown in Table 3.8.

Unfortunately the two surveys rate differently. HLS uses a four-point scale, the GHS a three point one. This could account for why the HLS respondents seem to be more optimistic about their health than do the GHS respondents.

Table 3.8 Self assessment of health

	Women					Men				
	Exc.	Good	Fair	Poor		Exc.	Good	Fair	Poor	
HALS respondents over 65 yrs	19	45	27	10	n = 936	23	44	25	7	n = 679
GHS respondents over 65 yrs	–	38	37	25	n = 2090	–	44	35	21	n = 1436

Source: HALS 1987; own analysis of unpublished data

Another explanation is that the HLS asks the respondents to rate their health 'for someone of your age' whereas the GHS does not. A smaller study by Cockerham et al. (1983) similarly asked, 'compared to someone of your age, how would you rate your health?' This changes the question from a self evaluation of health to a comparison with other older people. Cockerham et al. found that the older people in their sample were more likely to think of themselves as being in better health than their peers than any other age group. They related this positive assessment of health in older people to two factors. One, they claimed, was due to the fact that the older people saw themselves as survivors, the other that they do not have to maintain a high level of functioning and so their health is good enough to meet their everyday needs. This would fit with the belief explored in Chapter 2 that good health was being able to carry out one's normal activities. But a conclusion they do not draw is that older people are of the opinion that most other older people are not maintaining a high level of functioning and that they themselves are the exceptions. The implication is that they have internalized the negative stereotyping of old age although it does not match their own experience (Evers 1985). This relates to the views expressed by Williams', Wenger's and Thompson et al.'s respondents (Chapter 2, p. 31–2) Indeed one of the main reasons why Thompson et al.'s respondents did not feel old was because they equated old age with ill-health: 'They look on each other as old! And yet remarkably, scarcely any of them "feel old" or "think of themselves as being old"' (1990: 120).

Qualitative studies are full of examples of those who claim to be in good health in spite of chronic illness and disability. Clare Wenger (1988: 14) tells of one typical example from her study:

> Margaret Pritchard told me that she was in very good health, adding, 'I've got lots to be thankful for'. Her right knee was swollen to twice its normal size and she rubbed it as we spoke. When I asked about her knee she said it was 'just one of those things, you know, sometimes better, sometimes – (she left the sentence unfinished) – It's arthritis I expect, isn't it?' She had not bothered the doctor because she felt that this was inevitable at her age and that there was probably not much he could do. Subsequently, she told me that she suffered from colitis and tended to have diarrhoea in the mornings – 'no pain, just cramps'.

Table 3.9 Long standing illness or disability by self-assessed health

Self-assessed health	Has long standing illness or disability		No long standing illness or disability	
	Women (%)	Men (%)	Women (%)	Men (%)
	Well/ills		Well/wells	
Good	20	26	64	66
Fair	42	40	31	29
	ill/ills		ill/wells	
Poor	38	34	5	5

Source: GHS 1985; own analysis of unpublished data

In my own study (Sidell 1991) there were many similar examples. Naomi, for instance, who had terrific pain from her arthritic spine said: 'I'm certainly not an invalid. I just can't move otherwise I'm fine. No I'm not "ill" ill'. And another 94 year old woman said

> I'm really extraordinarily well, except that I fall about, cut my head the other day, had to have five stitches in it, but it really didn't upset me very much, I've had very good health. I've had various operations, this and that but I've always pulled through very well.

Given that in terms of the objective measures presented above, about 40 per cent of all those over 65 have no chronic illness or disability, then many of those who rate their health as good are doing so in line with objective measures. At the other end of the spectrum there are those who do assess their health as poor, again in line with an objective assessment of poor health. But apart from what might be termed the 'ill' ill and the 'well' well, there are those who claim to be in good health in contradiction of the objective measures.

Cross tabulation of the 'self-assessed health' variable with the 'chronic illness and disability' variable in the GHS data indicates the numbers of well/well and ill/ill and therefore also the anomalies, the well/ill and the ill/well. Table 3.9 shows this cross tabulation.

Various explanations of the anomalous categories of well/ill can be derived drawing on the exploration of health beliefs and attitudes explored in Chapter 2. There are those who publicly claim to be well but privately admit to be unwell – who feel that the acceptable public answer is to minimize health problems as identified by Cornwell (1984) and Wenger (1988). But some significant nuances in this public/private dichotomy can also be identified. There are the 'closet' unwells who actually deny their ailments in order not to be labelled old or viewed negatively (Wenger 1988). Then there are the 'relatively well' who consider themselves to be well in comparison to their own expectations of the health of 'old people' based on the prevalent negative stereotypes of old age. Lastly there is another identifiable group who are both 'healthy' and unwell. For them the two are not mutually exclusive possibilities because their definition of health is not merely the absence of illness but is a sense of 'feeling good'. Clearly they can have some form of chronic illness and still feel good. At the opposite end there are the ill/wells who have no chronic illness but do not 'feel good'.

We need then to be very wary of classifying older people as either healthy or diseased. The permutations and possibilities are many and are to a large extent dependent on the perspective of health which is held. Nevertheless older people worry about ill-health and the probability that they may have to cope with a chronic illness as they age. This is by no means inevitable and many older people do not suffer from such conditions. Also it is clear that many older people feel healthy with a chronic illness. Part 2 aims to explore the experience of chronic illness and try to discover how people maintain health in spite of disease.

PART II

Experiencing health

4

Understanding chronic illness and disability

Introduction

Illness presents a profound threat to the personal and social existence of the individual. When the cause of the illness is unclear, treatment a matter of trial and error, its trajectory uncertain and when the only certainty is that there is no real cure then it is indeed a 'mystery' that people survive. In this chapter we are going to review the insights and understandings of the impact of chronic illness on sufferers identified in what has become a substantial literature on the subject. The main purpose of this review is to provide a framework for the analysis of a number of case studies of older people living with both physical and mental chronic conditions. These case studies will be examined in Chapters 5 and 6 in order to discover how people do or do not manage to move towards the health end of Antonovsky's health-ease-dis-ease continuum.

How people survive chronic illness and disability has received some thoughtful attention within the social sciences, most notably by Anselm Strauss in the mid 1970s and more recently by Bury (1982, 1988b, 1991), Anderson and Bury (1988), Blaxter (1993), Charmaz, (1983, 1990), Pinder (1988), Williams (1984) and Radley (1989). Most studies are not age specific but because chronic illness is more prevalent among older rather than younger people the samples all contain a good proportion of older people. This literature is a rich source of theoretical and empirical knowledge on something which is likely to affect the health chances of many older people. All the studies aim to go beyond the biomedical perspective which focuses on the disease, its effect on the body and degree of threat to life, and move into the territory of psychology and sociology to explore the wider consequences and influences on living with a chronic illness. Bury and Anderson explain why;

> In a world of complex theories about factors influencing recovery and the course of disease (Kasl 1983), we remain relatively ignorant of the

everyday social, emotional, work, and family consequences of chronic illness. Little is known about the complex and sophisticated decisions made by patients and families to manage or control their illness through entering care, communication with professionals, or the management of treatment regimens.

(1988: 2)

Chronic illness is a generic term and covers a wide and diverse range of conditions. Much of the research focuses on one particular condition such as Parkinson's disease (Pinder 1988), the experience of strokes (Anderson 1988) or arthritis (Bury 1988b). But the issues with which they engage are very similar and common themes have emerged: the loss of self, disrupted biographies, the problems of finding meaning, dealing with uncertainty and unpredictability. There is a common concern with how people manage their chronic illness and the concepts of 'coping' 'strategy' and 'style' are explored by many of the researchers. Searching for answers to such questions as the following is common to most of those who find they have a chronic condition. What caused this illness? Why did it begin at a particular time? What is happening to me? What will be the outcome of this illness? What should I do about it? The relationship between the self and others is another strand in the work on chronic illness with the threat of social isolation being identified by many writers.

It is important to set the individual with a chronic illness within the wider contemporary society, both in terms of the available resources and the cultural values held, if we are to understand the complex interactions involved in living with a chronic illness. Modern western societies put a high value on competence (Bury 1991). Finding an alternative valued role can be tough for people with a chronic illness. Kathy Charmaz believes that:

> In a society which emphasises doing, not being, those who cannot perform conventional tasks and social obligations lose the very means needed to sustain a meaningful life.

(1983: 191)

Charmaz also suggests that people 'actively participate in their own discrediting' by internalizing the 'assumption that in order to be fully human, one must be able to function fully' (ibid.: 187). One of the most consistent attitudes to health expressed by older people in a number of studies discussed in Chapter 2 (Blaxter and Paterson 1982; Wenger 1988; Williams 1990) was that health was about being able to function adequately and to carry out one's normal daily business. It was considered a sign of moral weakness to give in to illness. How do people who hold such beliefs cope with their own chronic illness? In this chapter the insights and understandings of chronic illness which researchers have identified will be related to Antonovsky's (1984) 'sense of coherence' construct. Antonovsky sees the SOC as pretty much fully formed by adulthood, but it is by no means a static state and he is keen to stress its dynamic capacity. It seems to me that chronic illness tests, and poses a threat to, all three of the components of the SOC, comprehensiveness, meaningfulness and the ability to manage one's life. Making sense of chronic illness, coping with and managing one's life and finding meaning in one's life are essential if one is to move nearer to the health end of Antonovsky's continuum.

First a word about the terminology used to describe chronic illness and disability. The World Health Organization (WHO) classified the terms disability, impairment and handicap which might arise with chronic illness in the following way:

- *Impairment* is defined as 'any loss or abnormality of psychological or anatomical structure or function'.
- *Disability* is defined as 'any restriction or lack (resulting from an impairment) of ability to perform an activity in the manner or within the range considered normal for a human being'.
- *Handicap* is defined as 'a disadvantage for a given individual, resulting from an impairment or a disability, that limits or prevents the fulfilment of a role that is normal, depending on age, sex, social and cultural factors for that individual' (WHO 1980).

These classifications, although not unproblematic, have the virtue of being in current usage, most notably by the Office of Population Censuses and Surveys (OPCS). They are therefore useful for statistical analysis. But the meaning of chronic illness, disability, impairment and handicap for the individual who has to live with it is likely to be much more complex. Making sense of chronic illness to the sufferer is often a constant struggle. Finding answers to the 'Why me? Why now?' questions involves the sufferer in a complicated exploration of cause and effect and retrospective searching. The 'unfolding' and 'emergent' nature of chronic illness has been explored by Bury (1991) who points out that chronic illness by its very nature is not a one-off event, it is an experience which develops over time and one which has an uncertain trajectory. This puts meanings at risk because the situation is constantly changing. What the illness means now is not necessarily what it meant last month or will mean over the next few months. Consequently people are constantly engaged in negotiating and renegotiating the meaning of their situation.

The search for meaning

Bury has identified two types of meaning. One is meaning as 'consequence', the other is meaning as 'significance' (Bury 1988b). Meaning as consequence refers to the effects the chronic illness has on the lives of the sufferers. This may involve living with pain, discomfort and immobility. The illness may result in financial difficulties, loss of a job, the need to move house or become dependent on others. Establishing what the chronic illness means to people in terms of its effects on their body, their minds and their social situation is important if they are to be able to manage and adapt to these changes. Meaning as significance refers to the connotations that the illness has for people. Here the meanings are culturally significant and different illnesses have different significance, but almost all are a threat to the individual's competence and the significance of becoming an invalid, and therefore being 'in-valid', is invariably accompanied by the threat of social stigma and discrimination.

Ruth Pinder (1988) studying the effects of Parkinson's disease on patients points to the different significance the making of a diagnosis has for doctors and for patients. It represents a crucial turning point for both doctor and patient but in very different ways. For the doctor it represents an achievement, perhaps the end of a search for the meaning of the collection of symptoms presented by the patient. He/she has been able to name it. But for the patient Pinder claims, 'diagnosis may mark a day when life changes'. Their whole lives are plunged into uncertainty because the diagnosis rarely provides a clear indication of what will happen to them. Reactions to being given a firm diagnosis are likely to be ambivalent because,

> whilst the diagnosis of the disease provides something firm to relate to, and to explain to others, the actual nature of the disease remains elusive and the treatments empirical.
>
> (Bury 1982: 173)

Both Pinder and Bury describe patients' reactions to being told they have a specific chronic illness as being a mixture of fear and relief. Relief comes with knowing that there is something specifically wrong with them — they have not been imagining their symptoms and they can now prove this to others. But there is also fear because the doctor cannot tell them what to expect, how much pain or immobility is likely, how quickly the condition will deteriorate and what to expect of treatment.

The fact that most chronic illness has no known cause or cure means that medical knowledge is incomplete and the future course of events is at the mercy of trial and error. The limitations of medical science to provide an explanation for the condition they have can leave the sufferers with a complicated search for a cause for their own particular situation (Williams 1984). This is no simple quest for a cause but becomes a deeper search for meaning (Bury 1988b; Blaxter 1993). The illness is intricately bound up with the who and why of the person, their self-hood and personal biography. In Chapter 2 we explored people's beliefs and attitudes to health and illness in a general sense when they were without disease. When people are trying to interpret their own chronic illness they are trying to achieve 'experiential coherence' (Pinder 1992) which is much more complicated. They engage in what Blaxter describes as uncovering 'chains of causes' (1993: 137). In her recent re-examination of the data from the study of mothers and grandmothers referred to in Chapter 2, Blaxter explores the personal accounts of the grandmothers who were actually experiencing some form of chronic illness. She found that a feature of their accounts was 'the strain to connect, to present a health history as a chain of cause and effect, with each new problem arising from previous ones' (Blaxter 1993: 137). These chains of causes could go back generations and therefore become part of a familial or hereditary causal explanation. Both the 'connecting up of events of their lives' and the 'fondness for familial explanations' Blaxter sees as a need to establish continuity which enabled them to give meaning to their present lives with chronic illness.

Gareth Williams (1984: 177) believes that this process of establishing causal events and making connections between the illness and events and reference points in the past is a form of 'narrative reconstruction' which is engaged in to 'establish points of reference between body, self, and society and to reconstruct a sense of order from the fragmentation produced by chronic illness'. This narrative reconstruction serves not only to establish a causal connection to the illness but it also has a 'purposive or functional component'. It represents an attempt to 'imaginatively reconstruct' the past, to understand it, so that the present makes sense and has meaning and purpose. Medical knowledge and current thinking on the aetiology of particular chronic illnesses may be interwoven in the narrative but also discarded if it does not help to make sense of personal experience. This narrative reconstruction is not a once and for all account. The uncertain trajectory of chronic illness and its unpredictability require constant reconstructions of the narrative if chaos is to be kept at bay.

In terms of Antonovsky's 'sense of coherence' thesis these narrative reconstructions represent attempts to achieve 'comprehensibility' to

> perceive the stimuli that confront them as making cognitive sense, as information that is ordered, consistent, structured, and clear – and, hence, regarding the future, as predictable – rather than as noisy, chaotic, disordered, random, accidental, and unpredictable.
> (Antonovsky 1984: 118)

The 'purposive' and 'functional' component of narrative reconstructions is to achieve meaningfulness. It is the meaningfulness component which is particularly vulnerable with chronic illness.

The assault on the self

Kathy Charmaz from her qualitative study of 57 chronically ill persons concluded that the suffering involved in chronic illness not only entailed great physical pain and psychological distress but also a fundamental 'loss of self'. She found that ill individuals frequently experienced 'a crumbling away of their former self images without simultaneous development of equally valued new ones' (Charmaz 1983: 168). Bury's term 'disrupted biography' also describes this assault on the self 'where the structures of everyday life and forms of knowledge which underpin them are disrupted' (1982: 169). This is a consequence of the loss of meaning discussed above where taken for granted assumptions and behaviours are disrupted and common sense no longer makes sense.

Ironically with chronic illness it is the inability to separate the disease from the self which renders the self so vulnerable. Bury (1982) draws our attention to this more positive aspect of the biomedical model of health which objectifies the disease and separates it from the self. He sees this as a powerful cultural resource, one which legitimates illness behaviour and abdicates responsibility for the condition. But the nature of chronic illness makes this separation virtually impossible in that it pervades all aspects of the person's life. Added to this the failure of modern medicine to treat and cure chronic illness puts the onus back on the sufferer to manage the condition.

The individual with a chronic illness has not only to reconstruct the past to find meaning but also has to re-recognize him/herself and reconstruct a present biography and viable everyday life as well as re-examine future hopes and plans. This process of reconstruction has to take place within a context of uncertainty and unpredictability where the sufferer cannot count on his/her body to do the things which it was accustomed to do but where also even these limitations are constantly fluctuating. Anxiety, loss of self-confidence and loss of self-esteem are the frequent attendants of chronic illness (Bury 1982, 1988b; Charmaz 1983) making the reconstruction of a valued self a daunting task. Charmaz identified four ways in which the self is under assault because of chronic illness; by having to lead a restricted life, by being discredited, by social isolation and by becoming a burden to others.

Leading a restricted life

The terms impairment, disability and handicap imply that everyday life is restricted and limited and the normal activities that a person expects to be able to perform are no longer possible. Scales have been constructed such as the GHQ (General Health Questionnaire) and the Barthel Index of ADL (Activities of Daily Living) (Mahoney and Barthel 1965) which aim to test the severity of the disability and measure handicap. These scales record the person's ability to perform the tasks of daily living such as the ability to wash, bath, or dress oneself, cut one's toenails or other taken for granted personal tasks. But these scales do not measure the impact on the self of not being able to perform these tasks and the loss of self confidence and self esteem which can result from these incompetencies. Nor do they take account of the loss of freedom, pleasure and enjoyment from not being able to carry out previously valued activities. But the threat to self confidence and self esteem is compounded by the high cultural value that is placed on competence, independence and individualism. The Protestant ethic is at the core of many people's beliefs and attitudes to health and illness. This was identified by Williams and others and explored in Chapter 2. It can lead to ill individuals blaming themselves for their chronic illness as Charmaz points out:

> many ill persons themselves hold ideologies about living with chronic illness, which reveal residuals of the Protestant ethic . . . Chronic illness becomes the arena in which these values are played out. Maintaining a 'normal' life or returning to one becomes the symbol of a valued self. Under these conditions, chronically ill persons not only view dependency as negative, but also often blame themselves for it.
> (Charmaz 1983: 169)

In her reworking of the *Mothers and Daughters* data Blaxter (1993) explores the issue of why the victims blame themselves. She was particularly interested in how the working class grandmothers in that sample dealt with the notion of class inequalities in health because, although acknowledged by sociologists and social commentators, this was not an explanation for ill-health which they used. She concludes that they acknowledged deprivations in the past but they believed that these indeed were 'a thing of the past' and that people were now much better off and had little to complain about. She explains:

> They were perfectly capable of holding in equilibrium ideas which might seem opposed: the ultimate cause, in the story of the deprived past, of their

current ill health, but at the same time their own responsibility for 'who they were'; the inevitability of ill health, given their biographies, but at the same time guilt if they were forced to 'give in' to illness. With this emphasis on selfhood and self-responsibility, and their knowledge of greatly improved general social circumstances, a rejection of ideas about (contemporary) 'inequality' was understandable.

(Blaxter 1993: 141)

Nor do they question the 'normality' of ablebodiedness. Social life is organized on the expectation of ablebodiedness and only in the last two decades has this been challenged by those who are disabled. They have exposed the disabling nature of our society (Finklestein 1993; Oliver 1990). Those whose chronic illness and disabilities creep up on them in later life, who have identified and valued themselves as ablebodied are not part of what has become a supportive network of disabled people. They do not question the restrictive structures of society and so in many ways contribute to their own restrictions (Charmaz 1983: 174). But the handicap and disability which accompanies many chronic illnesses is difficult to adapt to precisely because it is so unpredictable. We have already discussed the limits of medical knowledge and the trial and error nature of treatment which contributes to this uncertainty. Added to this many chronic illnesses have long periods of remission when hopes and expectations are raised only to be dashed when the symptoms return. Sufferers also experience 'good and bad days' but the lack of reliability in the body means that people restrict their lives sometimes unnecessarily and find it hard to adopt appropriate behaviour in such changing circumstances. Restrictions on activities imposed by society and by the sufferer are a threat to the well-being, self-confidence and self-esteem of ill individuals, but perhaps an even greater threat to the self comes from the discrediting of chronically ill individuals.

Discrediting

Discrediting can arise from interactions with others as well as from within the individual who is frustrated and disappointed with him/herself because of the inability to function in ways that she/he would like. The stigma attached to visible impairments was identified by Goffman in his classic work on the management of spoiled identity (1963). He was operating within an interactionist framework and was interested in the ways visibly impaired individuals managed their interactions with others. Charmaz (1983) found that many of her respondents who had visible bodily changes due to arthritis restricted their activities rather than risk being discredited. Others limited their trips out and had to gear themselves up to face going out. But it was not only those with visible impairments who faced being discredited. Lack of competence and the loss of independence gave rise also to discrediting which could result in the individual being discounted. Although public awareness has been raised on this issue and most people are aware of the pitfalls of ignoring a person in a wheelchair and the 'does he take sugar' syndrome, Charmaz found many subtle ways in which her respondents felt discounted. This was particularly the

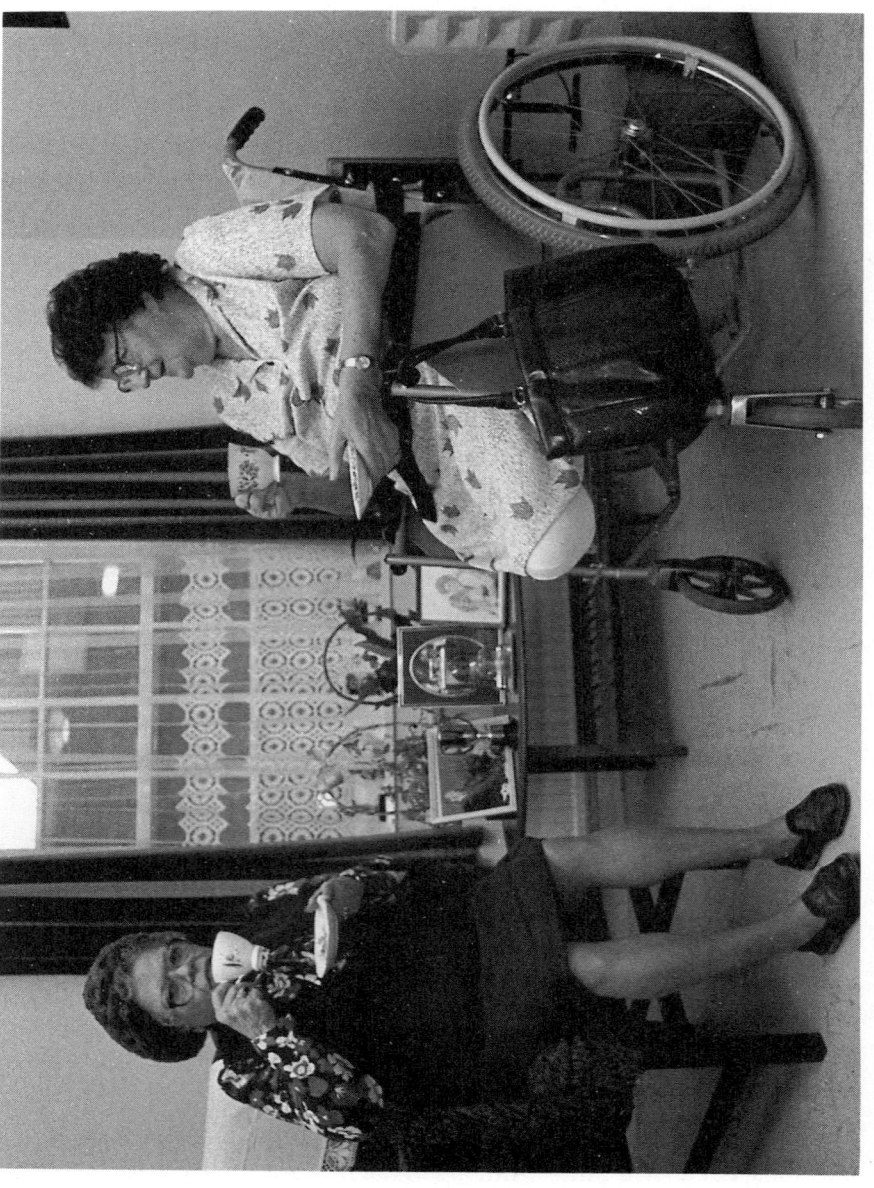

Enjoying a cup of tea together Photograph: Georgina Ravenscroft

case when their movements were slow or they had speech difficulties. Others would discount them by doing things for them or speaking for them.

Although all discounting and discrediting is hurtful to the self-image and damages self-esteem the significance of the discreditor is clearly important. Children in the street calling names is unpleasant but when valued colleagues, friends or intimates begin to devalue the chronically ill person then the threat to the self is much greater and further fuels the self-discrediting to which chronically ill individuals are prone. Conversely the continued support and affirmation of self-worth provided by intimates can help maintain the self-esteem of chronically ill persons. Personal relationships are very vulnerable to the strains imposed by chronic illness, however, and social isolation is a reality for many chronically ill persons.

Maintaining social relationships

A supportive social network is vital to the well-being of chronic illness sufferers, but chronic illness can test even the best of relationships. Bury (1988b) discusses how sufferers are wary and anxious about the effect the news of their chronic illness will have on those close to them. From his study of arthritis sufferers he found that this anxiety was greatest in the home. He describes how people would tell friends more readily about their condition, to test out reactions and gauge the effect of the news on their relationship. Whilst not minimizing the importance of maintaining friendships he found that with family the stakes are much higher. The sufferer is placing demands upon other family members and does not know what the limits of their tolerance will be. He found that rarely did spouses and other family members make a clear, open response to these demands and that the anxiety of both sufferer and supporters about the setting of precedents was high. The disruption chronic illness brings to the reciprocity in social relationships requires the renegotiation of pre-illness roles. People will be brought 'face to face with the character of their relationships' (Bury 1982: 169). Chronic illness alters the lives not only of the sufferers but also those close to them. Significant others are intimately involved in the chaos of chronic illness and their lives are likely to be restricted too (Anderson 1988).

Social isolation is a recurring theme in the literature on chronic illness and although those living with a supporter do at least have some interaction with another person, couples can be equally isolated. Withdrawal from social life because of immobility, lack of energy, embarrassment or preoccupation with the illness and its treatment is evident among sufferers (Strauss 1975; Bury 1982; Charmaz 1983; Anderson 1988) and this invariably involves the supporters, thus putting great strain on the relationship. Ruth Pinder from her study of people suffering from Parkinson's disease describes how couples are doubly isolated when friends and other family members do not visit because they find the proximity of chronic illness discomfiting. She quotes one woman who was looking after her husband:

> Friends, they don't *come* here very often. They phone me and tell me this and tell me that. But they don't actually *visit* here any more. They don't know how to behave towards him, I suppose.
>
> (Pinder 1988: 78)

Charmaz also comments on how shocked sufferers were at the withdrawal of attention from both family and friends.

The combination of the sufferer's own withdrawal from social life and the withdrawal of contact from friends and family can lead to loneliness and social isolation which compounds the distress of the chronic illness sufferer. But perhaps even more distressing and the eventuality most feared by chronic illness sufferers is that of becoming a burden to others.

Becoming a burden

Increasing immobilization results in greater dependency on others which is most feared by those with chronic illness (Wiener 1975). Dependency represents a final threat to a person's identity as power and control over their lives is lost. Some people feel acutely unhappy if they are unable to do their own shopping or everyday chores, which then have to be done by someone else. Charmaz points out that 'becoming a burden means that a person no longer fulfils the obligations implicit in past relationships' (1983: 187). She describes how ill individuals go to great lengths to contribute to household duties, feeling it is important to be useful in small ways at least. She maintains that the worst feeling of becoming a burden is that of uselessness and that this is intensified as the strain of caring takes its toll on the carer. Bury noted an interesting gender difference in the 'regression to dependency':

> Before the sick role is sanctioned men appear stubbornly stoical; once ill they show exaggerated weakness, a more open display of dependency being less structured in the case of women.
>
> (Bury 1988b: 108)

We have already noted that the values of competence, independence and individualism are strong in western culture and therefore this dread of dependency is likely to be strongest within this culture. Is it any less in other cultural traditions? Does the expectation that the family should cope with its older members make this less of a dread for Asian people (for example) who suffer chronic illness? Evidence suggests that for various reasons these values have been eroded amongst Asians living in Britain and the assumption that the family will care is not invariably a valid one (Bhalla and Blakemore 1981; Ebrahim 1992; Gunaratnam 1993). In general for all people suffering from a chronic illness it has been found that the fear of becoming a burden resulted in a heightened self-concern as the maintenance of everyday life becomes a major obstacle to independence (Charmaz 1983).

Although chronic illness is potentially devastating, in my own encounters with older people (Sidell 1986, 1991; Fennell *et al.* 1981) it was the way that they responded to the problems that chronic illness brought which was remarkable. It is only by acknowledging the full force of the threat chronic illness poses to the health and well-being of older people that we can really appreciate the very positive qualities they display in adapting to life with a chronic illness. I found that resilience, cheerfulness, adaptability, imagination, immense courage, robustness and humour were much in evidence. Miraculously people do survive chronic illness, they do overcome the obstacles although the odds are stacked against them. Bury believes that although some sociologists have been concerned with viewing 'people as agents' rather than the passive victims of whatever problems they face there is a tendency to be more interested in studying the problems people face rather than their responses to these problems. In the field of chronic illness the ways people manage their symptoms and treatment regimens was addressed by Strauss (1975) and since then Bury reports an 'accumulation of studies of the lived reality of chronic illness' (1991: 452). Whilst welcoming the attention paid to the ways people react to chronic illness Bury appeals for greater conceptual clarity and consistency in the use of terms such as 'coping', 'strategy' and 'style' which are those most frequently used to analyse how people adapt to chronic illness. Firstly, the issues involved in the management of symptoms and treatment regimens will be explored before going on to examine the concepts of 'coping', 'strategy' and 'style'.

Managing symptoms and treatment

Learning to live with chronic illness demands first a recognition of the symptoms before managing and attempting to mitigate the symptoms of the illness. The sufferer develops a new relationship to his/her body and an intense awareness of what it can and cannot do. Strauss described how:

> The sick person has to learn the pattern of his [sic] symptoms: when they appear, how long they last, whether he can prevent them, whether he can shorten their duration or minimize their intensity – and whether he is getting new ones.
>
> (1975: 41)

As well as this monitoring of symptoms the sufferer has to redesign his/her lifestyle to mitigate the symptoms. Sometimes this involves major changes such as moving house or giving up a job, but there are many other changes that people make such as buying clothes which are easy to get on and take off, taking regular periods of rest or being very careful to remember everything on a shopping list because popping back for a forgotten item may be a major operation. Again the unpredictability and changing nature of chronic illness makes this monitoring of symptoms and redesigning of the lifestyle a constant and time consuming activity. Strauss discussed how people with chronic illness and their carers become engaged in the daily management of time. Sufferers and supporters can become adept at 'temporal juggling' or the balancing of too much time or too little time. These temporal arrangements too are constantly disturbed by the changing nature of chronic illness. Managing the trajectory of the illness when it is so hard to predict requires a good deal of attention and fine judgement. Wiener used the term 'pacing' to describe how the people she studied, suffering from arthritis, identified 'which activities they were able to carry out, how often they could do so and under what circumstances' (Wiener 1975: 76)

A major part of managing the symptoms of chronic illness relates to the management of treatment regimens. We noted earlier that treatment for most chronic illnesses is still at the level of trial and error. So treatment is not simply a matter of compliance with medical prescriptions. Many treatments have unpleasant side effects and ill individuals have constantly to weigh up the costs and benefits of any treatment they are prescribed. Bury (1988b) noted how sufferers have to make decisions about the social impact of a given treatment. Strauss listed ten characteristics of treatment regimens which the sufferer has to weigh in terms of compliance:

1. Is difficult or easy to learn to carry out.
2. Takes much or little time.
3. Causes much or little discomfort or pain.
4. Does or does not cause side effects, especially if they are actually or seemingly risky ones.
5. Needs much or little effort or energy to carry out.
6. Is or is not visible to others.
7. If known, might or might not cause others to stigmatise the person.
8. Does or does not seem efficient.
9. Is or is not expensive.
10. Does or does not lead to increasing social isolation.

(1975: 27)

The decision to comply is not a once and for all one. As the illness progresses or new treatments are found so the sufferer will have to reassess the possible gains and losses. Many sufferers also make it their business to discover the latest treatments whether they are drugs or appliances. Seeking treatment, experimenting with it and constantly reviewing it, requires a good deal of 'both instrumental and affective "work" by patients' (Bury 1991: 459).

The management of symptoms and treatment regimens represents the practical response to the difficulties presented by chronic illness. The terms 'coping', 'strategy' and 'style' are used to analyse the ways that people respond to and counter the overall negative effects of chronic illness on the self and on social relationships. Although Bury accepts that empirically these concepts overlap, he feels that for analytic purposes they should be distinguished. He suggests that 'coping' refers to, 'the cognitive processes whereby the individual learns *how* to tolerate or *put up* with the effects of illness', (Bury 1991: 460) and it 'involves maintaining a sense of value and meaning in life, in spite of symptoms and their effects' (ibid.: 461). 'Strategy' refers to the actions people take '*what people do* in the face of illness' and 'the actions taken to mobilise resources and maximise favourable outcomes'. (ibid.: 462). 'Style' is a much less familiar term and perhaps more useful theoretically than empirically. Bury defines it as 'the way people respond to and present, important features of their illnesses' (ibid.: 462). Radley, who developed the concept in relation to married couples where the husband suffered from chronic heart disease, describes the concept as a 'style of adjustment' made within the terms of both social and bodily constraints (Radley 1989).

Normalization and the reconstruction of everyday life are two main ways of coping identified in the literature. Carrying on doing what is 'normal' was a definition of health identified in Chapter 2 and numerous commentators on chronic illness have described how sufferers strive to maintain their normal everyday functioning (Strauss 1975; Wiener 1975; Pinder 1988; Charmaz 1983). They do this by minimizing their difficulties and disguising their symptoms or by making superhuman efforts to overcome their handicap and carrying on as usual. When this is no longer possible they reorganize their everyday lives and reconstruct the taken for granted in an attempt to renormalize or construct a new normality (Anderson and Bury 1988, Pinder 1988).

Pinder used the concept of 'balancing' to describe a 'strategy' much in evidence in her study of people with Parkinson's disease. This involves interpreting one's situation and then making choices about the appropriate goals to be achieved and decisions about when and how best to achieve these goals. It inevitably involves trade-offs and as Pinder points out it is a social as well as personal process and involves bargaining with others, especially family. The changing nature of chronic illness means that this balancing has to be constantly redefined and new trade-offs made. As well as balancing pre-illness activities against each other another strategy adopted was to find new activities which were manageable within the confines of the chronic condition (Pinder 1988).

Two somewhat polarized 'styles of adjustment' were found by Radley (1989) which to some extent parallel normalization and the reorganisation of everyday life. 'Active-denial' was very much a style of carrying on as normal whereas 'accommodation' was more akin to readjusting personal and social life. Radley believes that the options open to people in terms of the style they can adopt are much less to do with the chronic condition and more to do with the social situation and the discourses available to people.

The overall manageability of a person's life conditions was the third component of Antonovsky's (1984) SOC and relates to the resources available to the person. The way people cope, the strategies and style they adopt do not occur in a social vacuum and clearly are, to a degree, dependent on the economic and social resources available to them. How personal and social resources impact on health and well-being will be explored in Chapter 7. In the next two chapters we are going to examine through individual case studies how people manage their own health and well-being. In analysing the case studies many of the concepts discussed in this chapter will be used to identify if and how people maintain health in spite of chronic illness. We will be asking how the individuals reconstruct the meaningfulness of their present circumstances and the 'narrative reconstructions' they engage in. We will examine the ways they manage their symptoms, their treatment regimens, their social relationships and the resources available to them. We will try to identify how they cope with the assault on the self, the strategies they use and the style they adopt to retain a sense of comprehensibility.

5

Maintaining health with physical illness and functional disability

The case studies which make up this and the next chapter explore the state of health of a range of individuals with whom I have been involved in the course of three research projects (Sidell 1986, 1991; Fennell *et al.* 1982). The case studies focus on the issues and concepts identified in the last chapter. Within each story the issue of how the individual makes sense of their health and illness and the meaning it has for them and for their lives will be drawn out. Their experiences with doctors and medical treatments will be explored as well as the changes they have made in their lives, and if, and how, they manage their illness. We will look at the effect the illness has on their social relationships, how they cope alone or with significant others, the strategies they adopt and their style of coping. These issues will be threaded into the stories and the purpose is to provide illustration and insight rather than representation. A comparative analysis will be made at the end of the chapter and this will be made within a framework of Antonovsky's salutogenic paradigm.

There are seven case studies in this chapter. We begin by exploring the situations of two people, a man and a woman, both in their late 80s who do not have a chronic illness or disability and who are very much in the 'well/well' category described at the end of Chapter 3. We then go on to look at three people who fall into the 'publicly well but privately unwell' category, a woman who is well *in spite* of her arthritis, another who is well *except* for her osteo-arthritic knees and a man with a prostate problem who is well but 'closely' unwell. Finally there are two stories told which belong in the 'ill/ill' category. One of these is a woman with arthritis, Parkinson's disease and bad varicose veins, the other a man who has had a series of strokes. The apparent inconsistency in the use of people's titles and first or second names is not arbitrary, but represents the degree of familiarity each subject invited.

Miss Hamish

Miss Hamish is 89 and very much a well/well person. She does all her own shopping, cooking and cleaning. She describes herself as 'fit as a fiddle, I've always been one for sports, cycling and skating and swimming and gymnastics'. She still walks a lot and swims once a week with an evening class. She has also attended woodwork and pottery classes.

Miss Hamish has a sister who at 91, apart from some arthritis is well. She has a brother in Devon who is 75 and apparently very well and her younger sister died at the age of 85. As she says they have mostly lived longer than their parents. Her father lived till he was 80 and her mother died at 66.

She is a modest person, almost shy but not unfriendly. Her hearing is not as good as it used to be and she has an NHS hearing aid. It is the type which fits behind the ear. She doesn't particularly like using it but does so when talking one to one with someone or when she watches television. But if she is in a group she finds that it does not pick up individual noises very well and everything becomes a blur. She has been tempted by the adverts for private aids that fit inside the ear but thinks they are a lot of money and is not sure that it will be that much better. She also had a period of bad eyesight before her cataract was operated on. This limited her activities and was not a happy period for her. She is very pleased with the cataract operation because it has restored her confidence again, which failing eyesight threatened. Recently she had a bad cold and so did not venture out as the weather was quite autumnal. She found this very frustrating and says that she dreads becoming housebound.

Her only complaint at the moment is 'itchy' skin which she says 'drives her silly'. She has been prescribed creams by her GP who is very sympathetic and has referred her to a skin specialist, but the tests revealed nothing. It seems there is little that can be done so she 'ladles' cream on to her skin and as she says at least it doesn't keep her awake at night.

Although not one to bother the doctor she nevertheless goes to the surgery if she is worried about anything and she feels that she receives good treatment; she has no complaints. She also regularly attends the chiropody clinic held at her local health centre and is very concerned to maintain her feet in good walking order. In all she seems to take very sensible precautions concerning health but does not engage in health promoting activities for health's sake. Her swimming and other activities are primarily for recreation and are part of her normal lifestyle. For her, health is very much about being able to carry on with her normal activities even though those activities may not be regarded by some as attainable at nearly 90. When asked to what she attributes her own good health Miss Hamish refers to her Scottish upbringing: 'Well it sounds absurd but I wasn't brought up to make too much fuss of myself. Scottish people, they are well even if they can hardly crawl about'. Her relationship to her parents she thinks was significant in other ways. They were devout Christians and in fact her father worked as an administrator for the church of Scotland. She describes her upbringing as 'narrow to a degree'. Her parents were very caring but her mother was particularly domineering: 'She sat on me, she was very overwhelming'. As a young woman Miss Hamish felt oppressed by her parents and needed to break away. This she did, she rejected them and their religion, which was like starting a new life. She describes herself as a strong person but says she felt stifled, especially by her mother.

She had been a schoolteacher all her life and had enjoyed working with children. She had never married due, she says euphemistically, to having been 'disappointed' in her 20s. In any case she thinks she would probably have been too independent. She clearly takes control of her life and does not leave things to chance. Typical was the way she decided and organized her present housing situation with which she is very happy. She lives in a sheltered flat in a privately run non-profit making old people's residential complex, with nursing home, residential home and sheltered flats all on one site. She made the decision herself and she chose the particular setting. She describes how

> I was getting on and I thought, well, I've got no one to look after me, and I thought about various places and I suddenly remembered Valley Homes. So I rang them up and said, do you sometimes take people who can't pay a lot? She said, write to me, telling us about what you've done, if we think you are suitable we'll keep in touch with you. So I wrote and they wrote back almost straight away, it was all done within three months. I sold my house and moved in and I did it on my own, I'm rather pleased with that. I made this decision, I was going to find a place, find somewhere. They're very small rooms, but it's my own flat. There's always someone available if I should need help but it's private and I've got my telephone, television too. And it's a beautiful outlook.

She has made new friends in the complex and gets on particularly well with one woman who is widowed. In fact far from losing her independence she feels that she has secured it. She is very contented:

> People say, are you happy? Happy is a very curious word isn't it? I'm content up here, I wouldn't be anywhere else, but the years that have gone don't get wiped out like that.

Being in control of her own destiny is very much part of Miss Hamish's coping strategy. She is of course an educated woman who is not without resources and she has a strong sense of her own capabilities. One of the saddest things she finds about being the age she is is that so many of her friends and contemporaries have died: 'my Christmas list gets shorter every year'.

Thomas Whiteside

Thomas Whiteside is a marvel; everybody says so. He is approaching his ninetieth birthday and has been widowed for nearly 12 years. He lives alone and does all his own cooking and shopping; he is fully mobile and can see perfectly well, although he has always worn glasses. He has no trouble with his hearing and he certainly has no memory problems. When asked to what he attributed his longevity and good health he would say, 'I don't know, I don't tek much notice'. If he could be said to have any philosophy at all regarding health it was not to make a fuss about it but to avoid worry; he believed that, 'worry kills you, that's what killed Jessie, she was a worrier, I used to tell her you'll alter nowt be worrying'. He certainly did not go in for any health promoting measures or change his lifestyle, but then he hardly needed to.

He lives in the same stone terraced house in a small Yorkshire town that he and his wife lived in all their married life and where they brought up their two boys. Both boys are married and live in the north of England but some distance away. His eldest son suffers much worse health than his father, having just had a mild stroke at the age of 59. He is a solicitor and fairly well off, in fact both sons have done well for themselves. The younger son had a much more varied career but is a successful businessman who has made a lot of money. Thomas was apprenticed from leaving school into the painting and decorating trade and had worked as a skilled tradesman all his life at the locomotive works which provided most of the employment for the men of that town.

He was never out of work nor off sick and although he did not earn a great deal they were a careful family. He didn't smoke or drink except for the odd sherry at Christmas and they ploughed all his earnings into the home and family. Both boys passed to go to the grammar school and although this was a state school and therefore they did not have fees to pay, they did have to support them into their early 20s. When one of them showed an aptitude for the piano they were able to buy him a piano and allow him to have lessons.

Thomas was born and bred in the town and has always lived within a half mile radius of where he still lives. One of his sisters used to live next door, the other in a nearby street. Both are now dead but he has a nephew and his wife who live up the road and two widowed nieces down the road. His father died in his late 60s from what Thomas calls 'dropsy'. His mother lived on well into her 80s and was a formidable woman. It is not clear what finally ended her life.

Before his wife died he had had to take over a lot of the domestic chores because she had bad arthritis. She in fact died of a heart attack and he didn't have to nurse her as such. After her death his sons thought that he would not be able to manage on his own either emotionally or practically. He had the option to go to live with either of them but he preferred to stay where he was. He had always been a very homely, family man and preferred to stay in familiar surroundings. He had his allotment which he had had all his life and where he grew prize chrysanthemums, sometimes the size of footballs. Their house did not have a garden, only a back yard, but on the allotment he grew all his own vegetables including tomatoes in the greenhouse. At 89 he still tended the allotment but someone else did the heavy work for the use of some of the land.

He showed very little overt emotion over his wife's death and seemed to get on with his life much the same way as he always had done. As he said, 'you've just got to get on with it, there's nowt'll fetch her back'. Since her death he had got into a routine. He did his bits of washing on Mondays. The boys had for some time been paying for the heavier washing to go to the laundry and for a woman to come in to clean one day a week. She came on Wednesday morning. On Tuesday he walked down to the shopping centre which was about half a mile away. The town was hilly and Thomas's house was situated half way up a long steady incline. Walking to the shops was therefore downhill but coming back with a load was quite hard work. His niece Alice, who was in her late 60s always caught the bus back. Thomas walked both ways and Alice used to berate him for carrying his bags up the hill: 'she says I'm daft to lug them heavy bags up road, but I can't be bothered standing waiting for bus, I can be home 'fore bus many a time'. Alice thinks the real reason is because he is too mean to pay the bus fare. For some reason bus passes were not available on that route at the time. Thomas had always been careful with money and was loath to spend unless he felt it was absolutely necessary. His sons' wives used to urge him to buy himself new clothes but he would say, 'that'll see me out'.

On Thursdays Thomas always went for his dinner to Nellie and Lizzie's down the road and on Sundays he went to Alice and Harry's up the road for tea. He always arrived at five o'clock after he had been to the cemetery to see to his wife's grave and he always left at ten o'clock. Alice and Harry were 'church people' and Alice would go to a 6.30 p.m. service after tea, leaving Thomas and Harry to do the washing up. Thomas was not a church-goer although the Victorian gothic church was just across the road from him: 'them as goes to church are not all they crack on to be. There's plenty better as keeps away'.

Some years previously Thomas had had a bad attack of phlebitis which kept him in for about a month. Nellie and Lizzie and Alice and Harry between them looked after him, doing his shopping and making meals. His sons were embarrassed about this and tried to persuade him to stay with one of them but he flatly refused. In fact they were constantly trying to persuade him to live with one of them permanently but he was adamant 'I'm all right where I am, I'd rather stay at home'. Thomas was always keen not to impose on his nephew and nieces and in fact over the last year he had been a great deal of help to Alice when Harry started to show signs of dementia. Thomas would go and sit with him while Alice went to her evening classes.

Although born and bred in the town Thomas had no friends, his relatives were his only form of social contact. As a couple he and his wife had always 'kept themselves to themselves' and he preferred to keep it that way. A bunch of local old men used to gather on a street bench if the weather was fine but Thomas never joined them, he would just pass the time of day. He liked to potter about his house and his allotment and he liked television, in fact they had been one of one of the first people in the town to get a TV in the early 1950s.

Thomas took care that his life was as predictable as possible, his coping strategy was to minimize change and not to take risks. When he had his attack of phlebitis he did whatever his doctor advised and always took his medicine. He was a contented man not given to excess or strong sentiments and stubbornly independent. His sons were planning a nineteeth birthday dinner in a rather grand hotel for all the surviving relatives. He wasn't particularly keen on this saying, 'I don't know what they want bothering for, I'd rather stay at home'. He didn't talk about the future much but neither did he seem worried about the prospect of death. In typical phlegmatic fashion he would say, 'I expect I'll be here till I drop'.

Sarah

Sarah has arthritis in her shoulders. It is very painful but does not restrict her mobility too much. She finds it hard to reach up now and so cannot do her own decorating which irritates her. Sarah had a 'bad' second marriage, a 'wandering' man whom she eventually left, but like most things she seems to have taken this in her stride. Sarah, who is 67, came to London from Jamaica in 1960 to join her sister who emigrated in 1956. She came alone although she had two daughters, one aged 3 the other 5. Their father had died and Sarah's mother and other sisters looked after them. She sent them money and brought them to England on holiday when they were 10 and 12 but they did not like it and so did not stay. Sarah's ties with her family are very strong and she went back to Jamaica regularly until her mother died. Since then she has tended to go back for special occasions, like when one of her daughters got married. Her other daughter went to live in the USA. Sarah also has visited her and keeps in touch with her grandchildren. She managed to conduct these transatlantic relationships on a very meagre income. For 20 years and eight months she worked on the London buses as a 'clippy', a job she thoroughly enjoyed. Although the pay was not good she was very careful with her money and always put some aside for her family and to pay her fare to Jamaica.

Sarah lived on her own for nearly 20 years but re-married in 1979. She now regards this as a mistake and was divorced in 1987: 'I divorced because the man was no good, boils down to the fact he was no good'. She goes on to elaborate;

> He thought I had money and he wanted money and because he couldn't get it we couldn't get along. And he was always running around with women and he would come in drunk and make a lot of noise so I couldn't take that. I like to live in peace – I just take myself off.

She now lives in a one bedroomed flat on a very large council estate in Hackney. It is a fairly modern estate, built on the deck system. However, although the flats are well designed and well built, the estate is run down and the many walkways and alleys make it an easy target for muggers and the crime rate on the estate is extremely high. None of this seems to worry Sarah and she is very happy with her flat.

She gives the impression of being a very capable and self sufficient woman who has strong views on most things especially health and illness. Her theories are certainly not one dimensional. Health is about happiness and laughter:

> Good health ? Well I think good health is when you can laugh and make people laugh . . . you can still go about, the limbs are all right, and you can make somebody happy.
>
> If you get a really hearty laugh, when it shakes you, because I know I have laughs when I roll, and my friends, we roll on the floor; it really lifts you. Doctors, they recommend laughter – it does something to the heart.
>
> Sometimes I wonder I go along the street and people look so miserable. Anything I do I go into it in full. Whatever you do, enjoy it, and you'll be happy.

Much of her enjoyment of life she attributes to her faith. She believes she has gained an excess of strength from her God. However she hedges her bets by keeping an exercise bike in her living room which she uses both to exercise her muscles and to lose a little weight because she is aware that being overweight is bad for you. She is very conscious of diet and healthy eating patterns. She firmly believes that people are less healthy now because of the chemicals in their food and drink and she compares this to the diet in the West Indies:

> If you notice some of these older people, they are living to 110, the thing is that in them days they didn't have these chemicals. That's destroying the human body, you know these chemicals they put in food. You don't know what to eat .. I guess that's why there's so much sickness. The people in the West Indies, they live to such a good age, they didn't know anything about these chemicals. We always had pure, fresh food, lots of fish, meat and vegetables nothing was added to it.

Plain water, she firmly believed, was a great health giver:

> A lot of people do not drink water and I think most of ill-health tends from not drinking water. It sounds funny but it is true that if you have a car and you haven't any water in it you know what happens. Well it's just the same with the body. People have so much kidney trouble. They say they drink tea and that's all right but no you have to drink plain water . . . you ought to drink ten glasses of water a day . . . just ordinary water.

Sarah never drank coffee or tea except herbal tea but it was interesting that she had a water filter which she had seen advertised in a magazine.

In terms of her own arthritis she held a 'wear and tear' theory, and thought that the condition had been building up in her shoulders for quite some time. She recalled some words of her father's, that it's not the same day that a leaf drops in the water it rots, it stays there for some time. She was also fascinated by the relationship of symptoms to the cause of disease:

> when every time you've got a symptom, it's not that it's always happening here. It's somewhere else something has happened and it comes out here. A river, it's there, but when it's full, it has to run over, it can't always stay there. So the thing is if I have a pain in my hand there's some cause somewhere in the body, something is not functioning why I get that pain there, it has to come from somewhere.

Whilst Sarah never let her arthritis stop her from doing anything, believing that you should never give in to illness, she also never ignored any symptoms. She took herself every three months to her GP for a routine check-up and she had recently insisted that she have her shoulders X-rayed to find out the extent of the arthritic degeneration. She also demanded, and got, a course of physiotherapy which she was just about to start. Sarah believed that the NHS was there to be used – whatever you want you ask for it. However her GP had drawn the line at her request for a body scan to check if anything else was 'fermenting'.

> Everybody is aware that the killers are heart disease and cancer, and I said to this doctor one day, I would like a scan. She say, Why? I said, well, if you have a scan and anything is wrong, it can be taken in hand before. No, she

could not because we'll have to know what we're looking for. I really did feel cross within me

But Sarah is selective in her compliance with medical treatment. She was keen on the physiotherapy but does not take any of the medicines she had been prescribed in spite of the fact that the pain in her shoulders sometimes kept her awake at nights, she prefers her own remedies:

> When people take all these tablets it's rotting your system. What I do, I get up in the morning and turn on the hot water tap and soak the rag in it and put it on it, and sometimes I spray it when I remember and I rub it with olive oil.

She also has her own supply of fresh vegetables. A council housing estate is not the most obvious place to find a flourishing vegetable garden but Sarah's balcony contains just that, a small, but very productive vegetable garden. It is an astonishing sight. In four large concrete containers, each about a yard square, forming the outside edge to the balcony, Sarah grows potatoes, maize, onions, tomatoes, large marrows, melons, runner beans, leeks, carrots and many other vegetables, rotating the crop through the seasons so that she always has a supply of fresh vegetables. Her father, she says was a great cultivator and she seems to have inherited this gift.

Although Sarah takes care of her health almost to the point of hypochondria, her way of coping with her arthritis is to ignore it and minimize the pain and stiffness by carrying on as normal. She took on voluntary work with a local charity as soon as she retired and goes four days a week to help run a drop in tea shop for older people. She is also a very active member of her church and sings in the choir. She has many friends through these activities and although she lives alone and most of her family are abroad she is never lonely.

> I like meeting people, seeing people, I like being among people because when I retired my sister said do dressmaking. I said, oh no, I couldn't sit down at a machine all day. I'm like a bird, to be out in the air that's me, I like to be out.

Sarah sees herself as healthy; her arthritis is an acceptable part of the wear and tear of life and is well within the bounds of what she considers normal and it does not disrupt her normal way of life.

Mrs Smart

Mrs Smart is 78 years old. She has osteo-arthritis which has affected both her knees. The left knee was the first to be affected but gradually over a five year period both knees have become very painful, swollen and stiff. Mrs Smart is quite sure about what caused it. Twelve years ago she was knocked off her bicycle by a taxi when the driver opened the car door as she cycled past. She was sent flying across the road and the handle bar of the bicycle went into her left knee. She describes how it hit the bone and she believes that the osteo-arthritis must have set in then and has built up from there. The fact that she now has osteo-arthritis in both knees and the handlebar only hit the left one has not deterred her from her theory, she says that, 'It must go down one leg and up the other, because this other one is getting really bad now and disfigured'. Her trauma theory, she feels, is backed by medical expertise and firmly believes that 'the medical people say that the arthritis is started by a knock'. She was adamant that it was not in her family and says that it was her doctor who told her that it had been caused by the accident:

> They told me it was caused by the accident. I didn't think it would develop like this, I never dreamt, I thought it would just heal and that would be that, but you see it didn't and that was the cause of it. It sort of damaged the bone and course as it goes on and on I suppose it deteriorates.

Mrs Smart has been married for 55 years. She and her husband live in a two-bedroom council flat which is very nicely furnished and comfortable. They have been there for the last 20 years and are very happy in it. The only problem is that it is a second floor flat and has quite steep concrete stairs to climb from the street level. Inside the flat everything is on the level but they are both afraid that the time will come when Mrs Smart's knees will not let her get up and down the stairs and she will become housebound. Mr Smart is very concerned about his wife's condition and is a great source of strength and support to her. He is a fit and healthy man just one year older than his wife. He has taken over the household chores without making any fuss although she tries to do as much as she can. The couple both retired when he was 65 although Mrs Smart had retired from her main occupation as a clerk in the tax office at the age of 60 and then had taken up part time work in a canteen until her husband retired from the post office. Having worked all their lives they now have reasonable pensions and so are financially quite comfortable.

The Smarts have three children, two sons and a daughter. All are married and they have numerous grandchildren. The sons live in England but 15 years ago their daughter emigrated to Canada. This was a big blow to Mrs Smart and she says that she had a nervous breakdown at the time which took the form of very bad depression. They visited and spent nine months there when they retired but decided against settling there because of her sons and the fact that their own roots were in England.

They have until the last few years thoroughly enjoyed their retirement and have travelled abroad on package holidays as well as their trips to Canada. In fact they have been in the habit of taking a winter and summer holiday. But the last year they had not gone away because Mrs Smart had not felt up to it. She had begun to feel depressed and very tired. She had had various blood and urine tests which had eliminated anaemia or diabetes. The doctor said that there was nothing specifically wrong and had prescribed a tonic for her.

Mrs Smart had great confidence in modern medicine and was well satisfied with her GP who she felt was very good and was always willing to listen and to explain everything to her. In fact she pinned all her hopes on having both her knees operated on and being restored to full functioning. She had seen the relevant consultant who had told her all about the operation and she was on his waiting list, but that was two years ago and she was still waiting. This Mr Smart thought was the cause of her recent depression because the time was going on and she seemed no nearer to having the operation. In fact she had been told that the list was so long that she would probably have to wait till she was chairbound. As she said:

> They're not thinking about relieving the pain. There are some terrible cases. I know I'm fortunate, I can still just get down the stairs and up again but there will be a time I'm sure when I can't, 'cos I know sometimes how it gets very tight. I think that's really bad because it's better to do it while you have got some movement and everything because you will recover better. And I mean as you get older naturally you are not having the confidence, are you?

She was afraid that she would deteriorate to the extent that it would jeopardize her chances of making a good recovery from the operation and this was beginning to really worry her. She had been upset when she had been told that if she was prepared to pay £3000 she could have the operations straight away. The Smarts were quite comfortable financially but they did not have that kind of money. Anyway they were firm believers in the NHS and were outraged that they were discriminated against in this way.

While she waited the Smarts managed her condition very much together. Mr Smart had become an expert on the tablets she was prescribed and had read up about each one and he monitored the effects of any new treatment. She tended to take whatever she was prescribed and she concentrated on managing her symptoms. She was very keen to keep moving but was aware of her limitations and so would 'pace' herself. She found standing particularly bad and told how she would

> do a little then sit down and then get up and do a little bit more. When I sit about I get so bored with myself and yet I think it's no good because I can't get up, perhaps I'll do a little bit of dusting for a little while and then they get so stiff at the back and I have to sit down and I think 'Oh blimey got to sit down again'. I had to just adjust to it.

Recently she has found it harder to sit about because she describes what she calls having the jitters. She finds herself getting very restless and jumpy.

The Smarts have always been a sociable pair and belong to numerous clubs, most of which they still manage to get to. She has recently begun to compare herself to some of the very old people at the club: 'There are some in their 90s and all that you know and when you see how they get about and jigger around I think, oh gosh why ever am I like this and can't do it?' Mostly she seems remarkably positive about her situation and is determined to keep going:

> You've got to push, you've got to persevere, you mustn't give in, he did tell me that. And I do agree because there are times when I don't feel like going out because of the pain, then I think, oh I must go.

In fact walking is much more manageable than standing and if they meet friends when they are out shopping she has a little strategy to avoid standing and talking for long which doesn't draw attention to her condition; she says to them, 'Shall we go in and have a cup of tea? You know and then you can sit down and it's given you a break'. She also avoids hills as going downhill is particularly difficult because her weight is pitched forward.

Mrs Smart is also careful about her diet and tries not to eat acidic foods. She is a little overweight and is trying to cut that down because she is aware that this will help her recover from the operation.

During the last year her optimistic view of having her knees operated on and being restored to full health was being eroded and she is feeling less and less confident that this would happen soon enough. The operation is central to the way the Smarts had up until now coped with the condition. They comprehend it as a temporary state of affairs. The accident theory is also part of that coping strategy and the meaning they attach to the osteo-arthritis. It was due to an external, one-off event which was certainly not Mrs Smart's own fault and the condition is one which medical technology could and should rectify. In this way it is separate from her self and so does not threaten Mrs Smart's sense of self. Managing it has come to dominate their lives but while this had been a temporary matter they could cope reasonably well with it. It was only as the time was getting on and the success of the operation was being put in jeopardy that it was beginning to look more permanent and beginning to threaten their general health and well-being in more serious ways.

Jim Wilson

Jim Wilson says he's fine and he certainly looks fit enough, but his wife tells another story. Jim is 76 and about six months ago Mrs Wilson noticed that when she came to do the washing, his underpants had a strong smell of stale urine. She didn't take much notice at first then she realized that his trousers were also sometimes stained. She didn't like to say anything — he'd always been such a proud and fastidious man. Then one night he wet the bed and was angry with himself, blaming it on an extra half pint he'd had at the pub. When it happened a second time he stopped going to the pub, saying that he was developing a beer gut and that was bad for his health. Mrs Wilson feels that this is a real loss to him.

The Wilsons had retired to a bungalow on the outskirts of Norwich because their only daughter lived there with her husband and two children. Jim had got into the habit of going to the pub about two or three times a week. He had made friends with two other men of about the same age with whom he played darts and in the summer he played bowls for the pub team. This sometimes meant travelling to nearby towns for away matches. Mrs Wilson had been rather glad about this because when they first moved he had been very bored and she felt guilty because she had been the one who was keen to move so that she would see more of their grandchildren. He had been quite happy about the move but had found it harder to settle than she did. They were northerners and had found the Norfolk 'reserve' a bit hard to penetrate at first. They also moved just six months after he retired and he was finding it hard to fill his days. She describes the bowls club and the pub as a 'Godsend'. She often babysat for her daughter and was glad to know that he wasn't sitting at home on his own too much.

Now, however, he would make excuses not to go. It was winter and so he would say he preferred to stay in and watch the TV, which really surprised her as he had never been one to watch a lot of television. However all this came to a head because they thought he had flu. He'd felt unwell for a couple of days and stayed in bed. Then she found him in tears in the toilet and he confessed to her that he had not passed water properly for a good 48 hours – just dribbles and his abdomen was quite swollen and tender. She got the doctor who said it was almost certainly prostate trouble.

> He was quite cheery about it all, said it was very common in older men. He made jokes about it cramping his style and how he couldn't expect to carry on like a youngster. Then he went into great detail about what an enlarged prostate was like. I was quite embarrassed, I thought it was only women who had troubles down below.

The doctor arranged for a district nurse to come and pass a catheter which at least gave Jim some relief. He had to go on antibiotics because he had a urine infection. Then he had to go to hospital for tests. Fortunately his enlarged prostate was not due to malignancy and Mr Wilson was put on the waiting list for a prostatectomy. Once the infection had cleared the doctor said that he would probably be able to pass water normally if he drank enough, went to the toilet regularly, and made sure that it had all come away. Mrs Wilson was not very happy about the doctor's attitude, she reported that:

> He just said 'not to worry, if it gets bad again we'll pop another catheter in and you can pee in a bag'. Well that wasn't very nice was it? Surely he could see that all this was upsetting Jim. Perhaps he meant it for the best, I expect he thought he would jolly him along.

Jim doesn't want anyone to know that he has prostate trouble. He did not even want to tell their daughter but Mrs Wilson insisted because, as she said, she would notice that something was wrong although of course there wasn't actually anything to show for it:

> It's like he's ashamed of it but I say to him, it's an illness like any other, but I suppose you feel different with something like that and of course he's not really ill – if you see what I mean. I know he's going through it but he doesn't say much. I feel so helpless.

Nobody in fact needed to know but Jim seemed to withdraw into himself which worried Mrs Wilson; she was hoping that he could have the operation soon. The doctor was not exactly encouraging, in his usual cheery fashion and with a good deal of innuendo, he had said that they shouldn't think that the operation 'would make a new man of him anyway'.

Lily

Lily lives in a one bedroomed modern bungalow in a charitable housing complex for older people. She is 74 years of age and, in common with many other older women, does not just have one chronic health problem, she has three; bad legs due to varicose veins; arthritis in her right hip which she says is going across into her spine, and a Parkinson's tremor.

She has considerable pain from her arthritic hip, she cannot walk far and only manages to walk about the flat, although she goes out in the minibus occasionally. Her hands tremble and she has difficulty holding a cup of tea. She always lifts the cup and saucer together to try to prevent spillage, but even so she constantly soils her clothes. This is a source of great embarrassment and means that she avoids most social occasions and only maintains contact with one or two very close friends and her family. But most of all she complains of tiredness, a constant feeling of wanting to lie down and rest.

> I never want to do anything. All I want to do is lie on the bed . . . that's how I feel, that's being honest . . . it sounds lazy, but it's not laziness, I've just no energy. I feel as though my legs won't go.

She does her own cooking and housework, her daughter comes once a month to do a big shop and she gets things on the weekly minibus trip to the local shops. She says that the flats are easy to clean and she isn't as 'fussy' as she used to be. She makes herself do one housework chore each day; she will hoover one day, change her sheets another and so on, but it always takes it out of her, as she says 'all my get up and go is gone'.

She is not aware of any family history of arthritis or Parkinson's disease although her mother had varicose veins. It is her firm belief that her present ill-health is all due to stress.

> I think all of it is the stress of everything, I think it's come to sort of a climax now. I can't explain it, it's sort of come to a head and I think it's all the stresses have really wore me out, and I'm tired really tired now. I've had so much stress in my life I think that's what it's done to me, It's sort of drained me, I've nothing left. This trembling, I think, stress has brought a lot of it. Stress can cause a lot of things . . . you've probably got it but it sort of brings it out. Stress is terrible for people.

Most of the stress to which she refers is due to a very unhappy marriage. This was made doubly stressful because of her lifetime's involvement in the church. The shame of a broken marriage was almost as bad as the marriage problems. Throughout the 30 years of their marriage her husband had constant affairs which she tolerated because they had four children and divorce was against her religious principles. In the end when the children were grown up and he was living part of the week at home and part with his other woman, she insisted that he decide on one or the other and he chose to leave her. She describes how:

> It took me about two years to get over it. It was two years before I could go to church, I just couldn't bring myself to go in, but I did in the end, I went back to church, because it's my life really.

She was left on her own and worked railway gates which gave her a living and a place to live. But it was hard work and she had to be up through the night and in all weathers. In fact her husband died in 1974 and because they were not actually divorced she was legally his widow and had to bury him, which was traumatic for her.

They had moved about a lot throughout their married life because her husband was in the railway police. One of her daughters had managed to get the present flat for her near to where she lived, but about a hundred miles from the other daughter whom she sees little. She is still in contact with her sons but also sees little of them because they live a long way from her. She is very dependent on her daughter who lives nearby, but she has a husband with multiple sclerosis who is in a wheelchair, and so finds it hard to spend much time with her mother. Although the housing complex staff and other residents are very supportive, she feels lonely and misses her family, as she says, 'you can be lonely in a crowd, can't you? Everybody is lovely round here, kind and helpful, but it's not family is it?'

In spite of all this misfortune Lily tries to remain cheerful: 'I've always had a good laugh. I laugh at things . . . at some things I shouldn't', but, she confesses, 'I'm not always cheerful. Sometimes I have a little weep, on the quiet, nobody ever sees it. I keep that to myself. I think it does you good to have a weep, it relieves you.'

Lily has had very little medical help either for her arthritis or her Parkinson's tremor. The doctor she had before she came to her present home had prescribed tablets for her Parkinsonism which she had taken for two years and which stopped the tremor. When she moved, however, the new doctor told her she did not need them, that she was not ready for them yet. So she stopped taking them, the trembling returned and now she feels it all over her body. On one occasion when her arthritis was particularly bad she described her doctor's reaction,

> I had terrible arthritis, terrible pain, I was crawling about the floor with the pain, and I rang up to see if he'd come and see me. He said, no I don't want to come out just for arthritis. Tell me your chemist's number and I'll send you some tablets through the chemist. That's what he did; they won't come out.

She has pain killers for the arthritis and some cream from the doctor and is resigned to her conditions:

> You just accept them, don't you? You don't sort of get over it do you? You don't get better, so you've just got to accept them, and do what is best for you as regards treatment or anything else. Like my arthritis, he gives me cream, I rub myself with cream and sit on a hot water bottle, I do all sorts.

For Lily her illnesses did not represent a 'disrupted biography' as described in Chapter 4 because they were totally integrated into her biography in terms of cause and effect; they were the inevitable consequences of her life's experience and as such had to be accepted. Her main way of coping has been to reorganize her life to minimize her activities and to withdraw from company. Acceptance is her main style of coping. She has managed to remain fairly independent; her strategy is to achieve one piece of housework a day and to do the cooking and care for herself. Her expectations and aspirations are therefore fairly limited but she does like to read: 'I get the library books, the big print ones . . . I like a bit of romance . . .'

Mr Ronald Clarke

Mr Clarke is 73. Twelve years ago he had a stroke which left him paralysed down his right side. He made some progress initially with walking and began to recover some of the use of his right arm but over the last few years he has suffered a series of mild strokes which have seriously weakened him and left him with some speech impairment. He is now chairbound and totally dependent on his wife for washing, dressing and feeding. He recently had acute retention of urine and now has an indwelling catheter because it was felt that he was not strong enough to have the necessary operation to remove his prostate which was causing the problem.

His wife, a fairly fit woman of 68, is weary and very tearful a lot of the time. The worst development as far as she is concerned has been the fact that he had now become both physically and verbally aggressive towards her. She thinks that a lot of the problem is because he has difficulty in making himself understood. But her doctor says that he might be a little confused because the strokes may have 'affected the brain'. This is the doctor's reason for not trying speech therapy:

> They think he's too far gone but I'm sure if he could get the words out a bit better it would help, I try to see what he wants but that's very difficult then he starts to shout which doesn't help and sometimes he'll just lash out at me. That's got so I'm very jumpy.

He will not let anyone else do any of the intimate tasks for him so she has to do everything and, although he cannot move far, she is anxious about leaving him alone. She does leave him for a short while to do the shopping but she is worried all the time she is out:

> I rush there, just get what I want and hurry back, what I wouldn't give just to wander round the shops, do a bit of shop window gazing but you've got that feeling in your stomach, what if he falls out of his chair or something, I don't know, you can't relax.

The Clarkes never had children; they both worked in the boot and shoe factory and were looking forward to their retirement, to taking it easy and pleasing themselves. Then he had the stroke and he had to retire prematurely. She admits to feeling bitter and resentful sometimes towards him and sometimes towards the system which doesn't seem to be of any help:

> They said you could have a home help but what do I want with a home help. This is only a small flat I can easily get round it that isn't my problem. I just want some peace and I don't get any company, you know the companionship has gone. He just sits in that chair half asleep unless something's bothering him.

She has had social services round and the social worker suggested that he go to a day centre. He became angry and upset at the idea and so she decided that she couldn't cope with the inevitable battle.

When he had his first stroke they had been optimistic. He seemed to make a good recovery; he went for physiotherapy and was taught how to exercise his arms and leg:

> he really pushed, made himself do them exercises, kept himself moving and he was coming on, you could really see the benefit. Then he had another turn that set him back, he was ever so disheartened but even then he kept trying, he didn't give up. But this since that took away his speech

that's been a blow to him, he's gone right down and I can't see what's going to pull him out of it. He's given up if you will but then he seems to take it out on me, you don't know what to think.

They are both now more or less marooned in a small council flat with no prospects of any improvement in their situation. She cannot make any sense out of it,

> He used to be such a big man, not fat, but strong, the last person you'd think would end up like this. I know there's plenty in the same boat, but you never think it'll happen to you. We've always looked after ourselves, you know plenty good food, well with both of us working we didn't go without, and he didn't smoke, we did go down the club of a Saturday night, he liked his pint but never over the top.

Originally they had coped as a team, their strategy had been to work on his affected limbs and gradually bring back 'normal' use. Clearly they had had to alter their lifestyle, giving up work and taking early retirement had to be adjusted to. They had coped with that, it had been part of their attempt to get his body back to some level of 'normal' functioning. Their style of coping was not exactly denial of the illness but a determination not to give in to it, to fight its debilitating effects. But each setback had required further effort and adjustment. They had constantly to renormalize their lives until it seems that the loss of speech was an overwhelming blow. He had given up the struggle and she was at the end of her tether, feeling helpless and unable to cope.

Thinking salutogenically

In terms of Antonovsky's health-ease-dis-ease continuum Mr Clarke would fall decidedly at the dis-ease end. Thomas Whitehead and Miss Hamish would be located at the health end. The rest would be somewhere in the middle. But would they be differently located if the assessment of their health was based on their subjective view as opposed to an assessment based on the 'objective' criterion of diagnosed disease? Figure 5.1 locates the subjects of the case studies on the health-ease-dis-ease continuum, the top representing their subjective self assessed health, the bottom their objective health status.

Both subjectively and objectively Miss Hamish and Thomas Whiteside are firmly at the health end of the continuum. Sarah is more optimistic about her health subjectively as is Mrs Smart. Jim Wilson also gives a more positive subjective assessment of his health. Lily and Mr Clarke on both counts are stuck at the bottom of the continuum, but Lily has a degree of acceptance which makes her position less stressful than Mr Clarke's.

Miss Hamish and Thomas Whiteside both have a very strong 'sense of coherence' in Antonovsky's terms. His concept of SOC, which was discussed in Chapter 1, consists of three components: meaningfulness, comprehensibility and manageability. The SOC of Thomas and Miss Hamish has not been threatened by chronic illness. In different ways both have found meaning in their lives; Miss Hamish mainly through her work and friendships and through struggling to establish her own strong identity in relation to her parents;

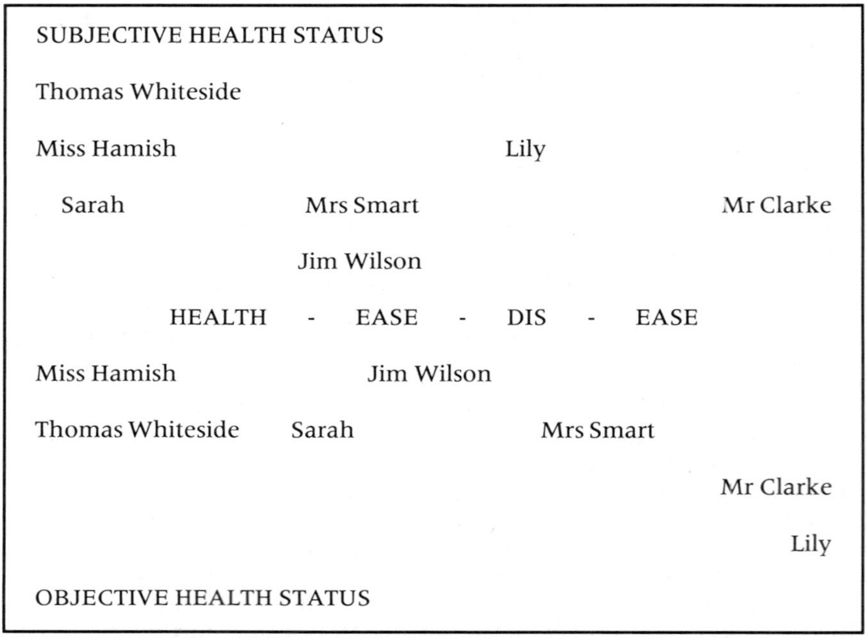

86 *Experiencing health*

```
SUBJECTIVE HEALTH STATUS

Thomas Whiteside

Miss Hamish                              Lily

    Sarah           Mrs Smart                        Mr Clarke

                    Jim Wilson

        HEALTH   -   EASE   -   DIS   -   EASE

Miss Hamish                Jim Wilson

Thomas Whiteside    Sarah                Mrs Smart

                                                Mr Clarke

                                                        Lily

OBJECTIVE HEALTH STATUS
```

Figure 5.1. The health-ease-dis-ease continuum: Objective and subjective assessments

Thomas through continuity and family ties. Predictability and consistency are almost the hallmarks of Thomas's character, he is determinably a man of habit and so his life is comprehensible to him. Miss Hamish's life is comprehensible because she feels in control of it. In terms of manageability both seem to have had neither under- or over-load problems in the demands made upon them. Both, in different ways, have participated in the decisions that have affected their lives; Miss Hamish by initiating and managing any change that she felt was necessary; Thomas by minimizing any change in his circumstances. Antonovsky is keen to point out that having a strong SOC is not necessarily admirable nor does it denote likeability. Thomas in many ways could be described as a rather irritating and ungenerous character and Miss Hamish a little self satisfied. But in health promotion terms the records of Miss Hamish and Thomas Whiteside are impeccable. Neither smoked or drank, and both took regular exercise although neither for reasons of health promotion. But although they are located firmly at the health end of the continuum this does not mean that they are totally without symptoms; as Antonovsky points out, no one is wholly healthy or diseased. Thomas has recently had phlebitis and Miss Hamish's hearing is not good, she has had cataracts and is very troubled with her itchy skin.

Sarah too has a strong SOC which her arthritis has not dinted. Her theories of illness causation have enabled her to make sense of her arthritis in such a way that it does not threaten her sense of self or in any way cause her to feel blame.

She has a sense of herself as a strong healthy person which she attributes to her faith; this gives meaning and comprehension to her life. She believes her arthritis is due to wear and tear and she manages it by taking sensible precautions plus whatever help she can get from modern medicine, but also by not giving in to it and by carrying on as normal and minimizing its effects upon herself. She locates herself very much at the health end of Antonovsky's continuum.

Mrs Smart has constructed a coherent narrative which enabled her to comprehend and find meaning in her osteo-arthritis and did not threaten her sense of coherence nor her relationship to her husband. She and her husband were jointly able to manage her condition because they construed it as temporary. It was on this basis that they coped. They renormalized their lives around it and they adopted strategies to mitigate its worst effects. Their style of coping was acceptance but only on a short term basis. Only as the chronic illness dragged on and took on a more permanent feel did it seem to threaten her sense of coherence and her ability to manage the situation. Their old style of coping and their strategies were not proving effective as time went on. From having maintained a position more towards the health end of Antonovsky's continuum she was beginning to move to the dis-ease end.

Jim Wilson also put his hopes on medical intervention but his style of coping with this potential threat to his sense of coherence was to accept it privately and temporarily but deny it publicly. His strategy was to withdraw from situations in which he risked exposure. This made it hard for his wife to give him the support that she felt he needed and in effect excluded her. It is very hard to locate Jim Wilson at either end of the health-ease-dis-ease continuum. Publicly he would no doubt put himself at the health end but his wife would probably locate him more towards the other end.

Lily would put herself at the dis-ease end of the continuum. She accepted her multiple chronic conditions and reorganized her life around them. Her strategy was to cut down her 'normal' activities to the bare essentials and then to put all her efforts into maintaining this restricted lifestyle. She had constructed a narrative around her illnesses which absolved her of blame and allowed her to redefine herself in terms of her illnesses. This was the way she coped and in some ways she managed to minimize the distress to herself and so managed to ease her situation. She had also been able to make peace with her church which gave meaning to her life. But her life had been difficult to manage and she had certainly experienced overload in terms of stressors and had not had a great deal of control over events.

Mr Clarke was very distressed and very much taken over by the cumulative effects of his strokes. Neither he nor his wife were now able to cope with their situation. They had exhausted their strategies and could find no meaning in their plight. His illness had destroyed his sense of coherence and the only style he could adopt was one of aggressive acceptance. This was destroying his relationship to his wife and posed a threat to her sense of coherence and ability to manage at all.

In the Clarke's case illness was a 'destroyer' in Herzlich's terms, or could be likened to Williams' category of 'illness as exile' where illness is controlled by 'normal' living; if normal living is seriously restricted then the person is finished, or they 'pass the time with distasteful alternatives' (see Chapter 2).

Williams' category of 'illness as disengagement' most clearly describes Lily's situation. This was a combination of 'illness as a loss to be endured' but also as 'a release from effort'. Lily was able to gain some relief from giving up and managed to do this without self-reproach because she attributed the illness to the stressful events in her life which were not her fault.

Sarah was definitely someone who saw illness as something which should be controlled by normal living and Mrs Smart was someone who saw her illness as a continuous struggle to maintain normality. For both of them in different ways illness was 'a test of achievement' (Williams, 1990; see Chapter 2). Jim Wilson's denial of his illness could be seen as 'illness as controlled by normal living' but in his case it is a pretence of normal living. In many ways he could be described as someone for whom illness was 'a loss to be endured' by forgetting about past interests.

In common with many older people identified in Chapter 2, most of the people depicted in these case studies held the strong belief that health was about carrying on normal living and that illness could be kept at bay or minimized by normal living. But there seems to come a point when this strategy is no longer effective. Time and the cumulative effects of chronic illness take their toll and determination and will power are no longer enough. Modern medicine was very important to them. Although chronic illness pervaded most of their lives and they drew on a range of explanations of health and illness, the medical model was the strongest influence on their management of their symptoms. All of them in their different ways depended on modern medicine as a strong plank in their coping strategies. The possibility that surgery would render them fit again was central to the Smart's strategy and possibly was what enabled Jim Wilson to deny his prostate trouble – it too was only temporary. A recognition that medicine could do no more for Mr Clarke contributed to their despair. Lily was disappointed in her approaches to her doctor and had accepted that nothing much could be done. Sarah on the other hand was determined to get all she could from medicine. She saw it an important resource in her armoury against disease. The doctor was also central to Miss Hamish's and Thomas's maintenance of good health.

None of the people depicted in these stories was entirely socially isolated, although as a couple the Clarkes had become isolated, and Jim Wilson and Lily were cutting themselves off from company because of the stigma they attached to their symptoms. The Smarts were consciously struggling to maintain their social contacts and Sarah's social life was central to her health and well-being. Both Miss Hamish and Thomas were less gregarious but nevertheless Thomas valued his family support. Miss Hamish had organized a support network for herself in the absence of family and was making new friends as the old ones departed.

In terms of financial resources none were overendowed but only Lily had experienced real financial hardship. Miss Hamish was the only middle class person, Thomas, Jim and the Smarts were all skilled manual workers with Sarah, Lily and the Clarkes in the unskilled category.

Many of the issues raised by these stories such as the personal resources available to older people and the social support networks as well as the implications of their dependence on the health services will be drawn out in Part 3. First the next chapter looks at the impact of chronic mental symptoms on the health and well-being of a range of individuals.

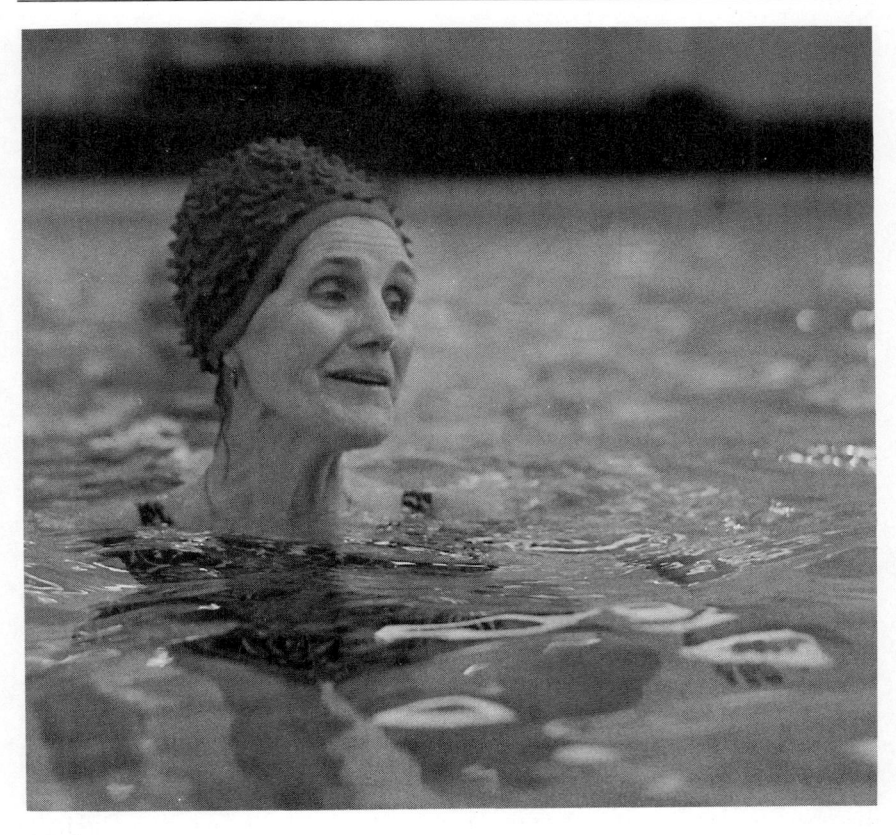

Splash
Photograph: Georgina Ravenscroft

6

Maintaining health with mental malaise

The literature reviewed in Chapter 4 on the impact of chronic illness related almost entirely to physical conditions. The separation of mental and physical symptoms is in many ways an arbitrary one, especially in old age where physical and mental problems coexist and in fact are often interdependent (Murphy 1988). However two mental conditions are of separate importance in old age to warrant closer examination. Depression, especially for bereaved older women, is something with which they frequently have to contend and dementia affects the lives of many older people either as sufferers or carers. In this chapter we will first look at the stories of two widowed women who have both experienced depression after the death of their spouses. One has managed to resolve her grief and reintegrate her life, reaching a state of wellness, the other still suffers 10 years later. The next story is of a woman who has spent two episodes in a psychiatric hospital suffering from clinical depression and anxiety which is not related to bereavement. There are three other case studies in this chapter all dealing with aspects of dementia. The situations of two men suffering from senile dementia who are being cared for by their wives and one woman who lives alone are described. As in Chapter 5 comparative analysis will be made at the end of the chapter.

Mrs Bernard

Mrs Bernard at 80 assesses her own health as 'not good at all' but she sees her health problems as mental rather than physical and much of her mental malaise she attributes to loneliness. She has been widowed for 10 years and has no children because she had three stillbirths due to rhesus incompatibility. Her mother died 10 years before her husband, with dementia. She was an only child and therefore has no surviving relatives. She never knew her father because he died the day after she was born from a heart attack.

Maintaining health with mental malaise 91

Her relationship to her mother and to her husband were both very close and loving and she misses them a great deal. She was brought up solely by her mother who did not remarry. She went to work in her mother's dressmaking business when she left school at the age of 14. She was clever at school and her teachers wanted her to stay on, but her mother said she could please herself and she chose to leave and work in the business. She did not regret this and thoroughly enjoyed the company of the two shop girls although her mother would have preferred that she keep her distance. After she married she did not work but visited her mother most days in the shop. Her husband was a skilled cabinet maker who always had work. They were not rich but comfortably off. After living in rented accommodation for a number of years they had saved up enough money to buy a small terraced house. They lived there for six and a half years until it was bombed in the Second World War and they lost everything. By this time her mother had sold the business and lived in a flat. After briefly living with her husband's parents, the flat next to her mother's became vacant and they moved into it (this is the flat that she still lives in). She was able to look after her mother when she began to lose her memory and she nursed her until two months before she died when she managed to get her into hospital. Ten years after that her husband died of cancer. Since then she has had a fear of doctors because her husband's cancer was discovered when he went for a check up on his eyes.

> Oh I'm scared of them. I'll tell you what started it. My late husband went to have his eyes tested for glasses. I went with him, I used to go everywhere with him we were so attached. Anyway when he got to see the optician he kept on looking at his eyes, he said 'Oh there is something wrong here' . . . so he said 'I would like you to see another doctor and have some tests'. Well it ended up with many tests, in the long run they found out he had cancer. Now that since has got into me and I don't want to go to doctors in case they find something. If you don't know then you don't worry, but if you do know then you jolly well do start worrying.

In fact she has had quite a lot of physical health problems over the last 10 years. She had two fairly mild heart attacks and was hospitalized for both and in fact enjoyed the company in the hospital. She has very bad varicose veins for which she wears an elastic stocking. This has affected her ability to walk far: 'Oh I'm so unsteady I can't tell you, I feel as if I'm wobbling from side to side. It's the weakness, the weakness in my leg that makes me wobble'. It was suggested to her that she use a walking frame but this idea did not appeal: 'Well how can you walk about with one of those things. It's so embarrassing, everybody looks at you, oh I would hate that'. Unfortunately she recently fell getting over the kerb and since then she has been afraid of kerbs. She is also afraid of the few steps up to her front door: 'I'll tell you I feel awful going up those steps, I hold on in case I fall'. This is due to the fact that her eyesight is bad because she has cataracts, her vision is completely blurred. She is waiting to have the operation but has been told it will be about six months. Although she would like her vision restored she is very frightened at the prospect and is trying not to think about it. She doesn't see herself as a healthy person and is quite surprised that she has lived this long: 'I'm amazed at myself that I've managed to live till this age, I always had this feeling that I wouldn't live to a ripe old age'.

It is not so much her physical symptoms that bother her but her mental state; she says:

> It's how I feel you know, I've always had that feeling that with me it was more mental than bodily, always thinking and thinking the worst, I'm always a one for worrying, I've got a worrying nature, I lay awake at night worrying about what is going to happen to me.

But she also describes more buoyant moods;

> You know sometimes you'd think I am ever so cheerful. 'Cos I'll have a mood and I'll start singing for no reason – I just happen to be and I can go through a repertoire I'll tell you, so many songs and so many tunes, not all English you know and I entertain myself that way till it wears itself out you know and that's the end of me.
>
> I can't describe it but if something nice and cheerful has happened to me I won't be so bad, but if you know it's the other way, oh I get so terribly depressed, you've no idea and it's due to the fact that I'm on my own.

The unpredictability of her moods bothers her: 'I'm not well because every day is different, no two days are alike'. Most of her troubles she feels are due to being on her own, 'not having a family, it's awful, you feel you don't belong anymore, you don't belong to anybody'. She still misses her husband and says she hasn't got over it; 'no you never do but, how can I put it, it fades a bit, I've still got pictures and a little miniature so I won't forget his face'. She regrets that they didn't mix very much 'when my husband was alive we were very reserved, we did everything together and didn't seem to need anyone else'. Consequently she does not have any friends and longs for company. She is looking into the possibility of moving into sheltered housing, but is overwhelmed by what she sees as obstacles in her way. The thought of organizing such a move she finds really daunting, especially the thought of dealing with all her possessions: 'A move appalls me, the thought of moving really appalls me, it's an accumulation of all those years, now I never throw anything out'.

She is a hoarder and her flat is cluttered in the extreme. As well as large old furniture the flat is crammed with all manner of things, an awful lot of which as she says is rubbish. There are piles of magazines, old newspapers, bits of material, books, clothes, plants in varying states of decay covering every available surface including the floor. In order to sit on a chair something always has to be moved and piled on to another chair. Everything gathers dust and there is a musty aura about the place. She is acutely aware of her untidiness and is too embarrassed to invite anyone to visit her because of it. This compounds her loneliness. She has a home help but because she does not want anything thrown away it is impossible to clean the flat and in any case she would rather use her home help's time to take her to the shops and to sit and talk over a cup of tea. Her home help is one of the few forms of social contact she has. In the absence of close and able relatives Mrs Bernard does not see how she could possibly negotiate and carry out a move.

She decided to try to arrange a holiday for herself and wrote to the council but as she hadn't heard anything and the summer was coming to an end she thought she had missed the opportunity and blamed herself; 'now I always leave things too late you see'. Mrs Bernard does not see herself as a capable woman at all and would dearly love someone or something to take charge of things for her. She is not a religious person but would love some metaphysical force to help her:

> All I want now is a voice which will give me help and I should be able to go on because I love life and I'll always want to do things or I think I will, although I don't think I do make the best of it you see.

She curiously manages to combine a good deal of self-deprecation with a marked sense of self-worth,

> You know I've got, not that I'm boasting about it, I've got an intelligence which is a little bit above the average you know, I understand things I do, I understand things a lot, not that it gets you anywhere but I think a lot and I realize things more than most people.

She sees herself as eccentric and different from other people. Although she is not happy with her lot she is not given to self pity nor does she give the impression of being a victim. Clearly she has had a lot of sorrow in her life but in spite of her situation she retains a refreshing enthusiasm and love of life and a sense of beauty: 'I love beauty in any shape or form, beauty, I've got a feel for it'.

Writing poetry is her way of expressing her feelings. When she is low in spirits she says 'I'll sit down and write a poem, I express my thoughts in the poem and then I don't seem to care'. She has at least a hundred scribbled on scraps of paper lying about her flat and she would dearly love to have them published. This one seemed to express her current mood very well. In Erikson's terms it indicates someone who has not achieved 'ego-integrity', but maybe that is because her aspirations are high; she is, as she says, a dreamer.

> Too late, Too late
> At times I like to take a look
> In memory's wide open book,
> page and page I carefully turn,
> there's so much there for me to learn.
> As in a dream my life goes by,
> at times I smile, sometimes I sigh,
> then I take a closer look
> at what I may have overlooked,
> to times when I would hesitate
> when I thought that I should wait . . .
> Sometimes when courage failed me
> and put an end to all I planned,
> I left undone what I'd begun
> Oh there was so much I might have done,
> this and that all gone amok,
> no more does opportunity knock
> now I feel that I have lied,

> I've let so much pass me by.
> Two words though I have grown to hate,
> too late my friends, too late, too late.

Writing is the way she copes with her wayward psyche but she is the first to admit that the rest of her life is a shambles. She would dearly love someone to take her over and reorganize things for her, but more than that she longs for human contact, to have someone close to share her life with. The cumulative losses in her life have been immense and this coupled with her physical ill-health, which she tends to dismiss, are a great threat to her well-being. Nevertheless she has a strong sense of self and is as joyful as she is dismayed by life.

Mrs Gerrard

Mrs Gerrard was 65 when her husband died four years ago. She was just beginning to feel well again. She had always since childhood had a 'weak' chest and suffered from bronchitis; she said it was in her family. She brought up four sons on a low income and admits to having neglected herself. She used to smoke until she collapsed with emphysema and because she lied to the doctor about her smoking she gave up immediately.

The boys were grown up and her husband semi-retired but working as a school caretaker when he died. They were living on the Suffolk coast. He had an operation for a stomach ulcer but it was found to be malignant. He lived for six months and Mrs Gerrard took care of him up until the last few days when his doctor decided he should go into hospital to give her a break. He went in on the Saturday and died on Monday. Although she was expecting it she found it to be a terrible shock in the end; 'you don't realise they have gone, even when they tell you'. It affected her very badly, she had been looking after him constantly and suddenly there was nothing.

She became very depressed.

> You are halved, your other half has gone, if you are young you would have your children to carry on for, if you are at work you would keep going but at my age you are halved, that part has gone, you will never get it back again.

She went to the doctor, was prescribed tranquillizers and was taking seven tablets a day. She didn't eat and lost two stone in weight. She describes feeling dazed and living in a fog.

Since becoming a widow she feels that she has toughened up. She did not think that she was a very strong person but she has had to 'grow another skin'. After her husband died she thought that things didn't go right for her and that everyone was against her. She found it hard to take on financial responsibilities because her husband had always taken care of them. She did not even know how to write a cheque. She describes going to the post office to get her widow's pension book:

> My heart was in my mouth, I asked for a form, I said my hubby's just died, I'm a widow, 'here's your form take it up the side and fill it in' he just give it

to me, he was ever so abrupt, I was shaking inside. People weren't perhaps unkind but perhaps I thought they were unkind

Building up her self-confidence has been a major task for her. Looking back over the period she has decided that most of her depression stemmed from the fact that she didn't cry when her husband first died. 'I thought I had to be brave for the boys, my eldest son said 'Mum don't cry, be brave, it will make us brave' which I did but that was wrong, I should have let it out'. She only realized this a good year afterwards. She was standing watching a remembrance day ceremony;

And I saw all these Air Force men and I didn't take no notice, I turned tail, crossed over the road and all of a sudden the tears came, the tears just came and came and came and I was so upset. That was Sunday. Then would you believe Monday morning I heard on the radio if you are bereaved you can go to CRUSE.

She found out where it was and went down there the next day; she describes what happened;

I walked in there and the lady said, 'come on you can come in there is another 2 ladies waiting'. She said 'what's the trouble?' Well I told her what happened on the Sunday, I said 'I cried and cried yesterday' and then I filled up, sobbed in front of her, so she said 'sit down and I will get you a cuppa'. And I sobbed and sobbed. I told her how I was on my own now since my hubby had died, I don't see much of the boys and how I've been so depressed and taking all them pills. That must have been playing on my mind and all of a sudden that burst. She said what it was all along, I should have cried.

Mrs Gerrard did not go back to CRUSE or have any more counselling. But she now had a coherent understanding of why she had felt so depressed and shaky.

The Jews they wail at the wall, Chinese bang drums, foreign people, foreign countries they always wail and wear black, even our royalty have six months quieter, not opening anything. With me that burst should have come right at the beginning, perhaps if I'd had a sister or a friend to cry with, but I had to be brave for the boys.

This understanding seemed to give her the energy and confidence to reassess her situation and she decided to instigate some major changes. She decided to move from the bungalow on the coast into a sheltered housing flat in Ipswich. She had not been able to keep the garden at the bungalow in good order and that worried her. Also she was rather isolated there. Although she didn't see a lot of her sons they all, except one, lived locally and always rallied round when she needed anything. They helped her to organize the move and physically moved her belongings.

The move also brought about another major improvement in her health and well-being. She had to register with another GP and her new GP was appalled at the medication she was taking. He gradually took her off all the tablets except one which she takes for high blood pressure. She describes this doctor as 'smashing, he sits and listens to you and makes you relaxed'.

She is delighted with how well she feels now. At 69 she says that she feels better than she did all through her adult life when she was bringing up her family. 'I feel lovely now, I feel like I was 18,19, yes I'm really pleased with myself, I got that inside me what I had when I was younger, before I had the family you know'. She works at keeping well. She has her own clearly thought out strategies. She takes care of herself medically by going to her doctor every month to have her blood pressure checked. If she gets any sign of chest trouble she goes straight to the doctor for antibiotics. She also takes cod liver oil and vitamins in the winter. However she is keen to point out 'I think of things first, I don't go rushing to the doctor, I study it first and think that will go away, I don't panic'. She certainly paces herself:

> Getting out of bed now I take my time getting out of bed, I can't rush, but once I'm dressed then I can turn the pace up a little bit, do a bit of dusting or what have you, then by eleven I think I've done enough.

She has made sure that her flat is easy to clean and has had wheels put on all the heavy furniture. She says that she has always been a great planner. She has now planned her life so that she doesn't get bored or lonely. She has joined clubs and loves her dancing club. She does anagram puzzles to keep her powers of concentration going. She has made a lot of friends in the sheltered housing scheme and visits and does shopping for some of those who are housebound. She has also worked out an evening routine as she is not particularly fond of the television. She always buys the local evening paper and carries out the following round:

> I get the paper and I shall read that by six, I'll take that up to Blanche upstairs, she will read it, I go up and have a little talk to her, then I go along the corridor to a woman I put drops in her eyes for her, she looks at the paper and then I take it to an old man upstairs. He's on his own, his poor wife is in The Elms [a Psychogeriatric unit], so I leave him the paper and he puts it through my door when he goes out shopping in the morning.

She doesn't allow herself to get worried about things and thinks that she can 'stick up' for herself better now. She is optimistic about the future, 'I think I will be independent now, I'm doing my own things and when my time comes I think my sons, they will help me'.

Having reconstructed an understanding of why she got into the depressed state she was in, Mrs Gerrard has totally reorganized her life and developed detailed coping strategies for maintaining her well-being. She has worked at creating a new identity as a widow from feeling that she had lost half of herself. This has taken her four years but if she had had a GP with a better understanding of the impact of grief instead of one who simply gave her tranquillizers, when her husband first died she might have reached that stage a good deal quicker. Fortunately she has encountered a more enlightened GP who has been a great ally in her management of her situation.

Laura

Laura is 66 and a very attractive married woman who lives in a large comfortable house in a leafy suburb of Norwich. In the last four years she has had two spells in a psychiatric hospital and is on lithium and amytryptaline. She describes herself as 'a very fit person, but I'm having a nervous breakdown, it hasn't gone away yet, although I've been discharged from the hospital, I have very bad days'.

It all started when she was about 62 without any previous history of psychiatric problems. She started to have 'funny dizzy spells or hot flushes' although she was well past the menopause. These were episodic and so she usually pulled herself together and got on with things. She went to the doctor and was prescribed pills for the dizziness and pain killers for a touch of fibrositis that used to trouble her. This went on for about three years until she became what she describes as 'unmanageable'. She went to the outpatients' department of the local psychiatric hospital and was treated with pills for about a month. But she got worse and became 'absolutely impossible, I couldn't sit still for a minute. I was banging my head and making funny noises'. She then became an in-patient and describes the hospital as 'absolutely marvellous'. She wasn't too keen on the case conferences but otherwise felt that the staff were very helpful and she got a lot of attention. The facilities were good; there was a gym, keep fit classes, yoga, dressmaking, cooking, pottery, woodwork and anxiety and stress management courses. But most helpful of all were the other patients. It was an acute ward and most of the patients were younger than herself, except for one man who was 70. She made some very good friends there who were very supportive to each other and she has maintained contact with most of them. But this has been also a source of disappointment to her because, as she says, 'none of them are really better'.

Laura was in hospital for six weeks and said, 'At the end of six weeks I felt really good, you know as though I could do anything'. But to her great dismay after three weeks at home she was back in again. She says, 'I didn't exactly go back to square one but it wasn't just an attack I had, it was two or three days and I was still bad for about a week'. She stayed in for about three weeks and since then has been going to the day hospital once a week. She also attends an anxiety clinic and is taking her medication. But she is bitterly disappointed that she is not cured. She said,

> At the time I thought, well, I'm cured now, I'm fine. After I'd been home after the first time, I got up one morning and I felt fine then I suddenly started to go down and I was really panicky about it because I didn't think it could happen. I went in the first time and I thought OK this is all over, gone. It never occurred to me that it could come back again. I felt so frightened because these moods although they're really awful while they're on, nothing happens, but you have the fears of things like you might faint, or you might fall over. The fear that I've got now more than anything is that I'll go completely irrational, mad is the expression that's usually used, but I'm too polite to myself to use that. That's the funny thing about this depression. When it's on you, you cannot see a future. You're down in this dark hole and you don't know how you're going to struggle

out of it. I really don't know what is going to happen because honestly I don't seem to be getting much better. I can put on an act now, I'm quite good at putting on an act. I don't know whether it's long term or not you see. I can go along quite happily and then something happens.

Laura has spent a good deal of time and thought on searching for a reason for her mental condition and trying to make sense of it. She recognizes certain triggers which are often related to anxieties over her children, particularly her unmarried son, but she tries hard to see some longer term explanation. Partly she blames her husband. Although their marriage was not bad in any dramatic sense – there was no violence or infidelity and they were a close family – she still thinks that,

> there was a certain resentment inside of me, a knot of resentment at the fact that he never really thought about me. When the kids were little he was never in the place, never in the house. It was typical of men of that era but I still felt it.

He was an accountant and had been a keen sportsman all his life and still played a lot of golf which kept him away from home a lot. She had worked full time after the children started school as a school secretary but she still ran the home and coped with the children. She remembers feeling constantly tired but as she said,

> All the time I was tired, I still carried on. I said to myself plenty of times, oh you can do it, you always have. I got into this rather frenetic way of living. I think that's got something to do with it. I don't want a frenetic way of living now.

She also describes how the first years of her retirement, before her husband retired, 'were the happiest years of my life', she felt free to come and go as she pleased, 'I really enjoyed myself I went and saw things, I joined things, and I saw plenty of my children and I really had a great time'.

Ageing has also had a significant effect upon her:

> One of the things that I think contributed to my being ill was the fact that I'd never accepted getting old. I'd always wanted to keep doing the things I did when I was younger. I just came to a full stop. I used to have all the kids up for a tea party on a Wednesday and it just got too much, you know and I couldn't think why. Of course it is that I'm running down, I'm not as young as I used to be. All kinds of things like that and it suddenly dawned on me, you're old and I couldn't take it at first. I'd never thought about it till then.

She thinks there might be some family tendency and describes her mother as 'highly strung' and can remember that she cried a lot when she was a child but there was no diagnosed depression. One of her sisters, had 'terrible depression' in her 20s but Laura thinks that this was post-natal depression. The sister got over this but suffered very badly from arthritis which Laura thinks might be linked to anxiety and depression. Her own acute bout of fibrositis she thinks was part of her anxiety.

The lack of a known medical cause and cure is a source of anguish to Laura.

She is pursuing various lines of treatment but with very little hope now after her initial disappointment. She is ambivalent about the medicines she is taking and her family think she should stop taking the pills but she feels that she can't expect the hospital to help her if she ignores their treatment:

> It's difficult to know because I'm very torn one way and the other. The hospital says take them because you're ill and when you're ill you have to take pills. I feel that in my hour of need I turned to the hospital and I think I'm asking for trouble if I don't do what they tell me, but I don't think they have done anything to help me, which seems to be borne out by the fact that I get better if I unburden my soul.

She is a very articulate woman and finds that talking through her feelings is a great help. The anxiety course was helpful and she has a counsellor whom she thinks has been of great value. One of the most effective forms of help, however, has been the two sessions of marriage guidance that she managed to persuade her husband to attend with her:

> We came to the conclusion that some of the cause of my illness was the fact that our relationship had got into a bit of a hole. We weren't really enjoying each other or particularly liking each other and we weren't being nice to each other, not very nice and so we thought that the best thing if we could get a counsellor and we did. He's been to two sessions. There's been a very different atmosphere since we went to the counselling, his attitude is altogether different. He realizes that it's a two way thing. David realizes that he should have been a bit more thoughtful and should have done a lot of things he didn't do, but I don't entirely blame him. It's ridiculous but you get sort of attitudes to people, I've discovered that all my life I've been doing things he's wanted to do, quite without thinking twice, and I've been fitting in. He's a fairly dynamic and fairly aggressive sort of person, dominating person so it's always been easier rather than have a row. Now, if I want to I can get him to do other things because he realizes that we've both made a mistake in the way we've been going on. He doesn't push me to do things I don't want to do.

This is quite a breakthrough and is particularly important because she feels very vulnerable and unsure of herself since this all happened and has lost a lot of her confidence. Although she felt safe in the hospital she is very much afraid of becoming dependent on it: 'I went back once and I didn't like going back. It makes you feel an awful failure if you go back again, I would really hate it'.

Going into hospital makes her feel guilty. She explains why:

> I've always been a coper. The last time I went into hospital I felt, what a weak person you must be. Well you're not in pain, you've got your faculties, you ought to be able to do things the way you always did but you can't, therefore you must be a weak individual that isn't prepared to have a go.

These feelings are very much related to her attitude to health in general which has been not to think about it, to just get on with things even if you are feeling tired, to ignore aches and pains. But she is finding it difficult to carry out this philosophy with her present condition, and this is leading to feelings of frustration with herself:

> The thing I've got to do is do things, steel myself to doing things instead of saying, oh I'd better not do that, I might not be well. But I've learnt not to do too much not to push myself too far. I need to build up my confidence.

It's the feeling that she cannot rely on her moods that makes her feel so vulnerable:

> I would like to feel safe in the situation I am in now and I don't feel safe at all because I never know when I'm going to have one of these awful breakdown attacks, and I don't really know whether I'm going to handle them myself.

This feeling of unpredictability in someone who has previously felt in control of her life is a blow, but Laura is trying to accept a somewhat different identity, seeing herself as vulnerable rather than strong and a coper. Her present coping strategy is to pace her life and renormalize her situation. This is very much based on the 'narrative reconstruction' of her life that she has engaged in to try to understand and make sense of her present predicament. At the same time she relies on medication to manage her symptoms but resists the label of madness and is afraid of becoming a 'revolving door' psychiatric patient.

Kate Cornford

Kate Cornford lived in a tied cottage in the Fens where she had lived all her married life. The cottage was some way from the village and so stood alone in the rather bleak fenland landscape. Kate was only 66 and physically very robust. Two years ago she lost her husband; they had no children. She and her husband had worked on the farm mainly dealing with the potato crop. After her husband's death Kate continued to work on the farm and a gang of potato graders took her in with them. Her failing memory led to inefficiencies which they ignored for as long as they could, but eventually, because they were on piece-work this began to threaten all their pay packets. Kate was retired but was allowed to go on living in the cottage and draw her pension. Many days she would cycle to work as usual and they would tell her as kindly as possible that she was retired now.

The farmer and his wife and other villagers became quite worried about Kate because she was often to be found wandering around the droves and dykes as though she was looking for someone. She would say that she was looking for Tom and nobody knew whether to remind her that he was dead or go along with the fiction and get her to go home. On one occasion a neighbour felt she ought to point out that Tom had been dead for some time but found that this distressed Kate a great deal. She had muttered, 'Oh dear, oh dear, I dunno, I dunno what's happening to me'. Coming to terms with loss and grief is difficult enough, but Kate was constantly having to experience this afresh. Facing up to the reality of his death and facing up to her own memory loss was clearly very painful.

Because they thought she was neglecting herself, some of the villagers took her into their homes for meals at the weekends and managed to arrange meals-on-wheels twice a week. Her GP arranged for a home help, a young woman from the village, who came officially once a week to clean. But Kate's memory and ability to care for herself deteriorated as did her ability to communicate. She would listen to what people said and she would start to reply but this would trail off into inaudible incoherent words. Similarly she would start to do something like make a cup of tea and then drift off somewhere else. Her home help came in every day to make sure that she got at least one meal a day and that the cat was fed – this was well beyond her official duties. The home help thought that she was desperately lonely and told how Kate would often put a few things in a bag and try to accompany her when she left.

Kate was always dressed for the land in an old sweater, trousers and wellington boots; she would wander aimlessly about looking quite bewildered. Winter was coming on and everyone in the village and the home help felt that they would not be able to provide enough support for her to cope with the cold. The only form of heat in the cottage was a Rayburn but Kate had long since lost the ability or the inclination to light it.

Kate was assessed by the psychiatric hospital who decided that she had definite symptoms of dementia, but she was not considered to be 'bad' enough for a psychogeriatric bed. Social services were called in and because there was no possibility of providing adequate support for her at home, Kate was admitted to a local old people's home. She settled in remarkably well and seemed very glad to be in the company of others. She did not wander or search for her dead husband and generally seemed relieved to be warm and cared for. She was able, with a little prompting, to care personally for herself in terms of washing, dressing and feeding and she had no problems with incontinence. She was pleasant and helpful to other residents and staff and rapidly became everybody's favourite. It is probable that had Kate's husband still been alive her dementia symptoms would have been quite manageable at home. She needed 24-hour social support, not to do everything for her but to provide cues and orientate her. Without that support her own home became alien to her and served only to remind her of her losses. The supportive atmosphere of the old people's home seemed to provide her with a much more secure environment and her health and well-being visibly improved.

Mr and Mrs Jones

Mr and Mrs Jones live in a three bedroomed modern detached house in an affluent suburb of Bristol. Mr Jones has been suffering from dementia for three years. His wife cares for him and he goes to a day centre for two days a week. Mrs Jones says that the onset of the dementia is difficult to date. He started to show an increasing 'slowness' but because he had always been a rather slow, ponderous man it was hard to know how worried to be. What really alarmed her was when he wallpapered the small spare room. He had always done the decorating and prided himself on meticulously matching the patterns on the wallpaper. This time he not only didn't match the patterns, he left gaps and wrinkles in the paper and didn't seem to notice. This worried her a lot. At the same time his driving became erratic and his reactions very slow. He put up no resistance when his daughter suggested that perhaps he shouldn't drive anymore and that maybe they should give the car to his grandson who was just learning to drive.

That was about a year ago and in that time he had deteriorated rapidly. He was now not capable of dressing, washing or shaving himself. He was unsteady on his feet and needed help with feeding. He was just continent but was increasingly having 'accidents'. Perhaps the worst thing was his regressive behaviour, although as Mrs Jones said that was better than him being aggressive and violent.

Because of his dementia their formerly very pleasant lifestyle had been eroded. They moved to their present house to be near their only daughter and her family 10 years ago. They had deliberately bought a house with a large garden because that was Mr Jones's favourite hobby. Now Mrs Jones employed someone else to look after it. Mr Jones showed no interest and did not even remember the names of the flowers that he had once carefully tended. Again she was distressed that he seemed to have completely lost all knowledge of something at which he had been so skilled. They used to be a very sociable couple and had attended the local church. Mrs Jones still managed to keep up her choir activities as their teenage grandchild came to sit with Mr Jones while she went to choir practices. But they had had to give up their regular weekly lunch outing with their daughter because Mr Jones's eating habits had become an embarrassment in the restaurants. Mrs Jones was also bitter that friends did not call round now because she felt they were embarrassed by Mr Jones's condition. It was important to Mrs Jones that he had a medical diagnosis and she was keen to point out to everyone that he had arteriosclerotic dementia, that there was an organic cause and he had not simply gone 'silly'.

Mrs Jones was very patient with her husband and never talked about him or for him in his presence. He did seem to follow parts of conversations and would put up his hand like a schoolchild if he wanted to say something. She would wait very patiently while he tried hard to utter a simple sentence and she was very adept at interpreting his thoughts and drawing him into any conversation. He seemed to get a great deal of pleasure from making these interventions. His granddaughter too was an expert in interpreting his needs and he was still very much part of the family.

He always appeared to be very contented and his sense of well-being seemed to spill over into his interactions in the day centre. Everybody there said what a 'gentleman' he was and how he was so well cared for. The two days that he went to the day centre enabled Mrs Jones to do her housework, visit her daughter in peace or simply rest. Nevertheless she was getting increasingly tense and had recently been experiencing a lot of headaches. Her GP was very sympathetic to her situation and had thoroughly examined her but found no medical cause. What really worried her was what would happen if she reached the point when she could no longer take care of him. Could she let him go into care permanently? She made a decision that she would only do this if he no longer knew who she was. For now Mr Jones was still a much loved and valued person.

Mr Jones's way of coping with his increasing incompetencies was to regress and behave in a childlike way. He was then able to take pleasure in small achievements like intervening in a conversation or making a crude clay model at the day centre. Fortunately, although this distressed her, Mrs Jones seemed to understand his need for praise and encouragement and was keen to preserve whatever competencies remained to him. She was not resentful or bitter, only sad that he was so diminished. It was vital to her understanding of his condition that it had an organic cause which she found acceptable and so did not have to reconstruct a narrative to explain his behaviour. The Jones's material and social situation was as ideal as one could hope for. They also had excellent medical support. Even so the health and well-being of Mrs Jones was becoming fragile.

Mr and Mrs Healey

It was hard to believe that Mr and Mrs Healey had both worked up to the ages of 79 and 78 respectively as chief waiter and waitress for a busy catering firm; they had run a car and often gone abroad for their holidays, including trips to South Africa to visit their only son. At 81 and 82 their situation was very different. The story is a familiar one. Mr Healey would go for walks and get lost. He was frequently brought home by the police. He had to give up driving because he kept driving up the kerb and couldn't negotiate the traffic. Like so many women of her generation, Mrs Healey had not learned to drive and so they lost the freedom a car had given them. He started to get up in the night and wander off. Incontinence became a problem. He also had a voracious appetite but would eat so much that he was sick.

Over the course of a year Mrs Healey began to lose weight and her GP sent her for tests to the hospital to rule out the possibility of stomach trouble. She was convinced that this was all a waste of time and felt that her lack of appetite and constant feelings of nausea were all due to nerves. She was very agitated about her husband's condition and although her own GP, who was different from her husband's, was very sympathetic to their situation, Mr Healey's GP just said that he was confused and would deteriorate and there was nothing to be done about it. His only suggestion was that she might 'try to get a Boy Scout to do her shopping for her'. Fortunately Mrs Healey's GP organized help from the social services who arranged for Mr Healey to go to a day centre for, first three days a week, then five. In addition the social worker spent many hours talking with Mrs Healey and absorbing her anger, frustration and outrage that nothing could be done to help her husband.

Relations between the Healeys were deteriorating rapidly. They had by all accounts been a reasonably harmonious couple. Mrs Healey had always been a bit domineering but Mr Healey had seemed content with this. Now he craved affection from his wife but she treated him brusquely and often unkindly. The main problem was incontinence, which she believed was deliberate on his part. He had become very unsteady on his feet and could only walk with assistance. He would ask to be helped to the toilet but when he got there he seemed to have trouble turning round and actually sitting down; consequently he would soil himself. She had given up taking him to the toilet to urinate and instead used an old saucepan so that he didn't have to move from the chair. Even so she was often too late to prevent him wetting himself. She would complain about this in front of him to anyone who called round and he would cry pathetically and say, 'I don't want to be like this'. She also complained that he would not let her sit and watch television. Apparently he would drum his hands on the chair irritatingly and always asked to be taken to the toilet when the news came on because she said he knew that she particularly liked this. He knew what was going on around him and in his own defence he would say, 'I want her to talk to me'.

Mrs Healey had, in desperation, taken to putting him to bed at 8.30 p.m. in order to get some peace. As a result he would wake in the night and call out for her. She now slept in the spare room because he wet the bed but had to attend to him constantly in the night. She had tried putting plastic pants on him but he would take them off and when she accused him of making a lot of work for her and keeping her awake at night he would say, 'I don't make a lot of work, I wouldn't do that, I'm a good boy'.

Apart from the social worker, Mrs Healey had no one to talk to. They lived in a council flat but Mrs Healey said that none of the neighbours 'wanted to know' since he had 'gone funny'. She was now putting all her efforts into getting him taken into full-time care but his incontinence was a problem for local authority homes and he wasn't supposed to be 'bad enough' for a psychogeriatric bed. His doctor thought that she was not managing the situation very well. It was certainly a very unhappy state of affairs. Mrs Healey was bitter and resentful, she could not make sense of his condition and could not accept his regressive behaviour. Both his and her health and well-being were deteriorating and there seemed to be no hope. She was not coping and had no strategies to deal with the situation. Unfortunately her social worker who was her only form of support was reluctant to call in too often because Mrs Healey had so much pent up anger that it was impossible to extract herself in under two hours and so she had to set aside a whole morning or afternoon for the visit instead of calling frequently.

Health with depression and dementia

Locating people on the health-ease-dis-ease continuum is much more difficult with conditions such as depression and dementia. Mrs Gerrard's health and well-being had dramatically improved in every sense both physically and mentally. Mrs Bernard's had not. Laura felt very unsure of her mental state although physically she was very fit. To an observer Kate's health and well-being seemed paradoxically to improve by entering residential care. Comparatively the Jones's situation was a lot 'healthier' than the Healeys. Clearly a whole range of factors can 'ease' both depression and even dementia.

The situation of Mrs Barnard was not eased and can best be described as one of 'desolation', the word used by Bernard Isaacs in the 1970s (Isaacs *et al.* 1972) to describe the extreme loneliness and isolation which some older people experience. And yet of all the people whose stories have been told in this and the last chapter she is the person who has the highest aspirations and she still experienced moments of great happiness. Well-being for her is more than getting about or doing one's normal daily business. She aspires to what Maslow described as a state of self-actualization, but her poem describes her despair that it is 'too late' to realize this – that she has failed to attain, in Erikson's terms, 'ego identity'. It is hard to find meaning in life now that she is alone and her life seems in disarray. Grief has destroyed her sense of coherence and without some form of help she has not been able to overcome this. Had she someone in her life on whom she could depend, particularly who could have filled the confidante role (Murphy 1988), she may have coped differently, but she is utterly alone and remains at the dis-ease end of Antonovsky's salutogenic continuum. In complete contrast Mrs Gerrard has found 'health' after a similar feeling of despair. She has sons who, whilst not being a source of emotional strength to her, have at least provided practical help which has enabled her to find congenial living circumstances. She managed to construct an account of why she became so depressed so she was able to make sense of her feelings. She was then able to rebuild her life and adopt coping strategies to make sure that she was not lonely. Her sense of coherence, although shaken had been thoroughly restored.

Laura's battle to find meaning in her anxiety and depression and to hold on to her identity has not been altogether won. She has intensively reviewed her life and her relationship to her husband and has reached some plausible conclusions. She has also developed strategies for dealing with the unpredictable and frightening losses of control that she experienced. Her husband has also had to re-evaluate his own behaviour and try to understand his wife's perspective with the help of counselling which indicates that marital counselling can still be effective even after 40 years of marriage. Although she has made progress in maintaining a sense of well-being she still feels vulnerable and is only fragilely coping. She is ambivalent about the help available from the health services. The hospital was a great help initially but the fact of having to return to it represented such failure for her that it is no longer a source of support. She does gain a great deal of support from talking through her feelings; she is unsure about the benefits of the medication but is afraid to dispense with it. Laura has a lot of social support from her family and she is the first to acknowledge that her general circumstances are extremely good. This in some ways has made it difficult for her to come to terms with her problems.

If any condition could be said to threaten the identity and break down any sense of coherence, it is dementia. It can mean many losses as well as loss of memory not least the loss of a sense of security. The study of dementia since the mid-1970s has generated a great deal of literature and the disease has made an impact on the public consciousness. Most work has focused on its aetiology, assessment and treatment. A lot of attention has been given to the plight of informal carers. Recent writers have begun to explore what it might feel like to experience dementia, but it is hard to get inside the experience of someone suffering from it. Kitwood (1993) has drawn out the potential for increasing the wellness of dementia sufferers through sensitive care and communication in either a formal or informal situation. He emphasizes the need for an 'other' to interpret and represent the 'self' of the dementia sufferer instead of assuming that it is irretrievably gone. Kate's sense of insecurity and incoherence was palpable. Her woebegone and bewildered expression and her inability to make sense of what used to be very familiar surroundings was clear to see. She had no 'other' to understand and interpret her needs. She must also have experienced grief at the loss of her husband and constant companion. She was not able to come to terms with this because the event was not fixed in her memory, and she constantly displayed the characteristic signs of pining and searching for her dead spouse. Paradoxically she was much more content in a residential home which was totally unfamiliar to her. She seemed to feel more secure where there were always other people and where she was warm and well fed. Perhaps she was experiencing the possible reassuring effect of what Kitwood has called 'a culture of dementia', where common bonds are built up between dementia sufferers who seem to manage to communicate with each other, often non-verbally (Kitwood 1993: 64).

Both Mr Jones and Mr Healey seemed to have lost their adult identity and regressed to a childlike state. Research in the Netherlands (Miesen 1993) has explored a similar state which is common in dementia sufferers, that of searching for a long dead parent, usually the mother. Miesen uses attachment theory to explain some types of behaviour seen in dementia. The idea is that some dementia sufferers, seeking security in an uncertain world, come to regard their carers as they did the main provider of security when it was vital (i.e. their mothers in infancy). Mr Jones and Mr Healey seem to relate to their wives as mother figures, perhaps to recapture their sense of security which they have lost from their consciousness. As a strategy, albeit an unconscious one, it seems to work better for Mr Jones than for Mr Healey. But then Mr Jones plays the good child, Mr Healey the naughty child. Although both situations are difficult, the Jones's situation is a good deal 'healthier' than the Healey's and Mr Jones seems to be more content than Mr Healey. In fact Mrs Jones fulfils the role of 'other' and her way of relating to her husband and especially her patient way of communicating with him, follows closely that which Kitwood identified as enabling dementia sufferers to achieve the four 'global states' necessary to reach a state of well-being; self-esteem, agency, social confidence and hope. She validates her husband's experience through her nurturing which manages to fulfil Kitwood's criteria;

> *A communicative act was carried through successfully.* The dementia sufferer felt recognized as a person: *self-esteem was enhanced.* A gesture was transmuted into action: *agency was confirmed.* The dementia sufferer moved towards the Other and was welcomed: *social confidence was increased.* Confusion and disorder within the psyche was met with order and stability in the social world: *hope was sustained.*
>
> (1993: 66)

Mrs Healey was not able to respond in this way. She blocked communication with Mr Healey and even put him to bed to distance herself from him. She no longer recognized him as a person and talked about him and over him in his presence. Her rejection of him diminished his self esteem and self confidence and there seemed little hope of relief for either of them. But Mrs Healey had no social support, and her husband's GP was quite unhelpful and sometimes hostile. The Jones's social circumstances were much better than the Healey's and Mrs Jones has a great deal of support from her daughter and family. If the

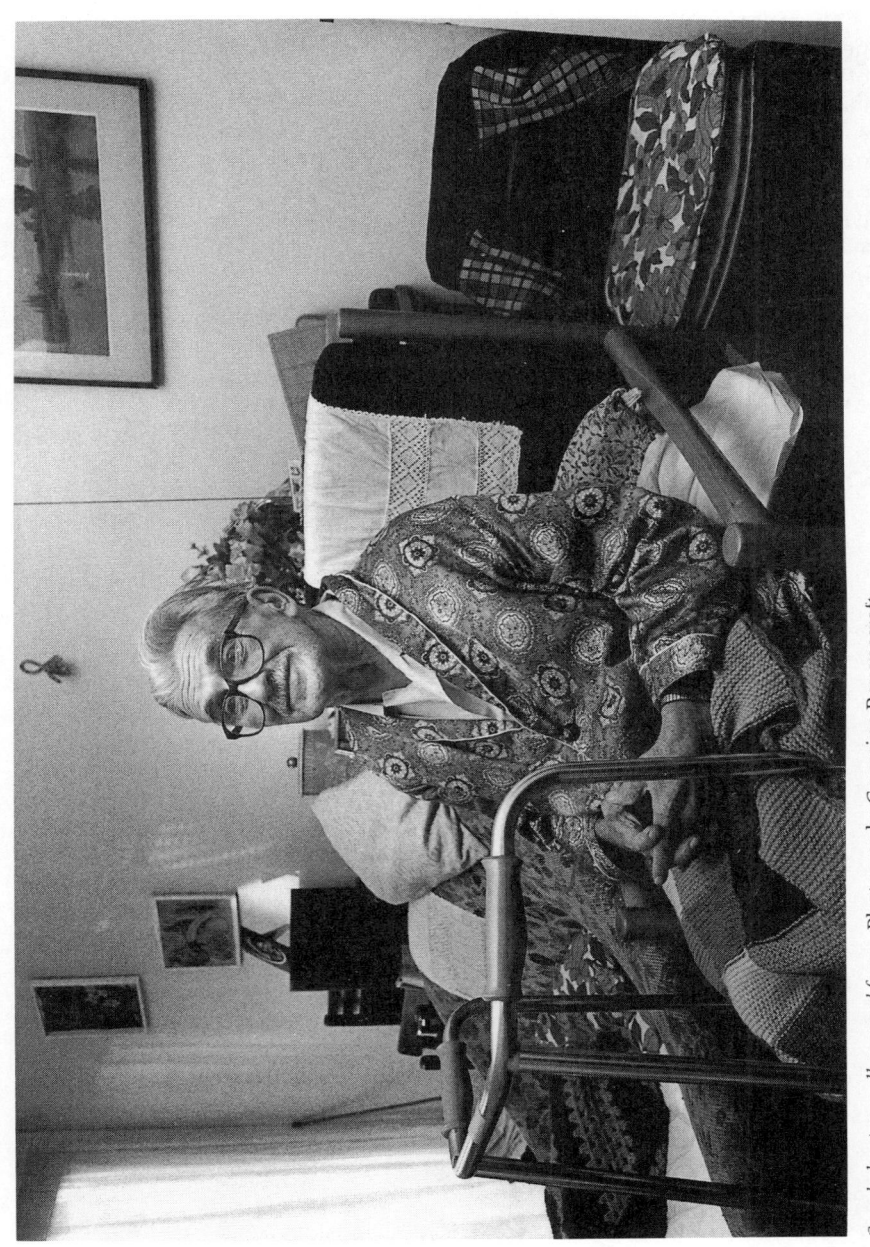

Cared about as well as cared for   Photograph: Georgina Ravenscroft 'other' is to adequately fulfil this role of proxy identity to dementia sufferers then the carers too need help and support.

There are many interacting factors which enable people to move towards the health end of Antonovsky's continuum. Many people maintain health in spite of chronic illness both physical and mental. The way they do so seems rather like negotiating a series of snakes and ladders. People climb to the health end by constructing a ladder of meaning only to slip down again on the snake of unpredictability, but they may then climb up another ladder with the help of social support or statutory health care. Situations are rarely static. In the next part of this book we will examine closely some of these 'snakes' and 'ladders' such as personal resources, social supports and health care and draw out the implications for public policy.

PART 3

Resources for health

7

Health care and the management of health

Most of the time people take care of their own health. Professional health services play a relatively small part in the management of an individual's health, but they are an important resource in the maintenance of good health and in dealing with disease and consume a large part of the national budget. In this chapter we will discuss the importance of the statutory services for the health and well-being of older people before going on to assess the level and scope of self-health care.

All of the people featured in the case studies turned to the statutory health services when they had health problems which were beyond their own resources to sort out. They had expectations of the health services but these were not always met and their opinion of the service they received varied a good deal. Whatever its shortcomings, the National Health Service (NHS) is extremely important to older people in the UK and any erosion of the services it provides is likely to be at the expense of the health and well-being of older people. What does it offer older people?

Aims and claims of the National Health Service

In Britain the NHS promises universal coverage of free medical care at the point of need. The aim is to provide an equitable service to all citizens wherever they live and whatever their socioeconomic circumstances. As such it claims to be a socialized service but critics have argued that in fact it is a nationalized rather than a socialized service because power has never rested with the consumer but remained with doctors and administrators (Doyal 1979). Nevertheless the conception of a state provided system of health care embedded in a wider welfare state has its roots in a more collectivist rather than an individualist ideology. Anne Jamieson (1989), comparing health and social care for older people in a number of European countries and the USA, puts Greece and

Denmark at opposite ends of the spectrum in relation to the ideological and political factors which underpin the provision of health and welfare. She places the UK nearer to the Danish model but notes the recent erosion of the principle of state responsibility:

> Historically, Britain has had a relatively comprehensive welfare state which has included a range of social services for those in need. However, the last decade has witnessed gradual changes in an attempt by a strong centralist conservative government to reduce the role of the state in funding and providing welfare. In spite of public opinion, which still predominantly favours public provision of welfare, the government is pursuing a policy of increased self- and family reliance, especially by restricting the budgets of local authorities, which are responsible for social services.
>
> (Jamieson 1989: 453)

Recent moves to care in the community can be interpreted as wresting power from the remote and expensive hospital sector and funding services at a local level theoretically more sensitive to local need. This results in a loosening of the ties of responsibility of the state to provide this expensive hospital care and making the community responsible for the care of its citizens. Unfortunately without a shift of resources to local authorities, responsibility for care in the community will fall on individuals and families. The danger is that the lack of consumer involvement in the NHS identified by Doyal (1979) can be taken up by a conservative government and translated into market terms resulting in a shift to consumer choice based on the ability to pay.

We will examine in more detail the implications of the community care legislation for older people later in this chapter. In terms of the NHS it represents a move of resources from the hospital sector to the primary health care sector. What has the hospital sector had to offer older people?

Hospital care

In the 1980s acute in-patient care accounted for about a third of the NHS budget. The NHS provides care within a medical model of health. The service is mainly curative with the emphasis on treating acute and particularly life-threatening illnesses and restoring the individual to a disease free state (Wilkin and Hughes 1986). Older as well as younger people have benefited from this acute medical attention but older people present problems for this type of service. As we have emphasized throughout this book the health problems facing older people, especially older women, are more likely to be chronic than acute and they encompass physical, mental and social concerns. There are broadly two consequences to this. One is that older people inappropriately take up acute hospital beds, the other is that the service does not meet their needs. Wilkin and Hughes argue that the specialism of geriatric medicine grew out of both of those concerns. The problem of 'bed blocking' by older people as perceived by acute specialists 'created a powerful force for a separate speciality' (Wilkin and Hughes 1986: 171), and in MacIntyre's (1977) 'organizational terms' (see Introduction) overcame the opposition to spending large amounts of money on a specialist service for older people. The motivation of Marjorie Warren, who is regarded as the pioneer of geriatric medicine, was rather different. She was working in the late 1930s and was convinced that with proper examination, investigation and treatment the physical condition of many older people could be improved (Evers 1983). Since the 1930s the speciality of geriatric medicine has developed to a very sophisticated level but as Wilkin and Hughes point out it has substituted rehabilitation for cure:

> Medical intervention in geriatric medicine operates on a continuum between dependence and independence rather than health and illness. The medical model has been shifted in the direction of a functional conception of health. In this way it is possible to achieve success measured in terms of patient through-put, which permits the speciality to claim, if not achieve, parity of status with acute specialities.
> (1986: 171)

The criterion of success is to raise the level of independence of the older person in terms of the 'normal' activities of daily living and as such is in tune with the view of health held by many older people that health is about carrying on one's normal activities. But it is also reinforcing the high value put by society on competence. In this climate, continued dependence is seen as failure both for the medical profession and for the older individual.

Acute hospital services, with their potential for saving life or fully restoring vital functions like sight through cataract operations or mobility through joint replacement surgery, are essential to the health and well-being of older people. The benefits to be had from the rehabilitative functions of modern geriatric departments should not be minimized. But, although consuming a large proportion of the NHS budget, the hospital service is used by only a minority of the population compared to the primary health care system provided by the family practitioner service.

Primary health care

Every British citizen has the right to be registered with a General Practitioner on whom he or she can call for free medical treatment. The GP also acts as a gatekeeper to a wide range of other services. As we will explore later satisfaction with General Practitioners varies a great deal and it is this variation in provision which is cause for concern. From a study of 200 GPs Williams and Wilkin (1988) found great variations in the patterns of care provided. They report an 'enormous' range in the way GPs relate to older people, the level of home visiting and the level of consultant referrals. They comment:

> While health and social services are striving to achieve uniformity of provision for old people, individuals living next door to each other can experience gross differences if they happen to be registered with different GPs.
> (Williams and Wilkin 1988: 40)

As well as differences in attitudes and approaches between GPs there are more definable differences in the facilities available. These range from small one or two doctor practices operating from lock up premises to large health centres with five and more GPs working with a range of other health care professionals such as nurses, social workers, chiropodists and physiotherapists thus providing a wide range of services. A further potential for inequalities in service provision lies in the ability of some GPs to become fundholders and to control their own budgets. How this will affect the quality of provision to older people is hard to tell at present but there is anxiety that GP fundholders could be deterred from accepting large numbers of older people onto their lists because this may incur larger than average expenditure.

Another development in the provision of primary health care to older people is the introduction of the new GP contract which came into effect in 1991. This requires GPs to offer a health check to all those over 75 years. The following broad list of categories for the health check is offered as a guidance in the contract:

1 Sensory functions
2 Mobility
3 Mental conditions
4 Physical conditions, including continence
5 Social environment
6 Use of medicines

There is the potential within this for taking a much more holistic and social view of health and as such it is to be welcomed, especially as the contract stipulates that the client should be offered a discussion of the results of the consultation and therefore opens up the opportunity for greater exchange of information. A review of the use of medicines is also to be welcomed.

From the feedback on the early workings of the contract it seems that the lack of statutory guidelines is allowing for wide variation in interpretation (Barker *et al.* 1992). It could be that instead of ironing out the differences in care provided by GPs this could be reinforcing it. GPs who have always practiced good care for old people will diligently carry out these checks, neglectful GPs will get round the requirement. Some pensioners' groups fear that the extra workload that the health checks impose will cause some GPs to discriminate against older people, that they will be reluctant to accept the over 75s onto their list. Already many older people find it hard to change their GP which, given the great variation in the care provided, is the only safeguard they can have (Cooper, Scalter and Sidell, forthcoming).

The case-finding aspect of the health check should go some way to redressing a balance which has long been identified as a deficiency in the health care system, that of preventative care. There is evidence that older people are discriminated against in screening programmes (Henwood 1990a). Routine screening stops at 65 for breast and cervical cancer in women despite the fact that 40 per cent of deaths from cervical cancer occur in women over 65. Women over the age of 65 are routinely screened for breast cancer in Sweden, the Netherlands and the United States and studies have shown that it is cost-effective (Fletcher 1992). While screening for breast and cervical cancer has been the subject of a great deal of attention and public debate, screening for cancer of the prostate in men has received much less attention, maybe because it is a disease which affects mostly old men. Of all cancers diagnosed in men 13 per cent are of the prostate and 8.6 per cent of all cancer deaths in men are due to this disease. Yet, if identified at an early stage surgery and radiotherapy can be effective. Advocates of widespread screening for cancer of the prostate claim, drawing on evidence from a small number of screening programmes, that it is cost-effective, can identify a large proportion of early stage cancer and prolong survival time (Chadwick et al. 1990). Those opposed point out that the incidence of cancer of the prostate increases enormously with age and that about 30 per cent of all men over the age of 50 and 90 per cent of men over 90 would show evidence of cancer on histological examination. They also point out that as men get older they are more likely to die from other causes and so aggressive treatment would be unwise and result in unnecessarily worried men and a great deal of overtreatment (Schroder 1993).

The value of screening procedures in general is in doubt because they can be intrusive and generate feelings of anxiety (Freer 1985; Taylor et al. 1983). The case finding approach seems more appropriate to the needs of older people where wider health problems can be identified which threaten the ability to function as well as the general well-being of the older person. Taking account of the social environment and the social support available and including the older person and their life history in the analysis of the problem and possible solutions would be more in line with the 'biographical' approach to the assessment of need in older people advocated by Gearing and Dant (1990). Much will depend on the approach to health taken by the GP. If he or she takes a strictly medical perspective then the health check will do little more than root out yet more high blood pressure. If the GP takes a more social and holistic view of health then there is scope for improving the health and well-being of older people. But is it realistic to expect GPs to carry out what would be a lengthy and time consuming procedure? And is it the GP's job to be involved with what are more social matters? The division between health and social services has always been an artificial one, particularly in relation to older people and it is one which the 1991 NHS and Community Care Act goes some way to bridge.

Community care

Older people's health needs straddle the traditional health and social services boundaries. This has implications both at the budgetary level and at the professional and organizational level. In budgetary terms it has created inequalities in the system and inappropriate and inefficient care. MacIntyre (1977) argued that community care has always been sold on both organizational and humanitarian grounds (see Introduction). There are certainly good arguments for breaking down the organizational and professional fragmentation of care in relation to older people. In an atmosphere of diminishing resources it is tempting to pass responsibility for individual older people onto the other service. By defining a problem as medical or social each agency can transfer responsibility onto the other. In a study I conducted with 'confused' older people (Sidell 1986), this was very apparent. Some old people were actually shunted from one service to the other with very little regard to their health and well-being. Assessments of the same older person's level of confusion would differ considerably depending on who was making the assessment. Hospital personnel would claim that the person was 'too good' for a psychogeriatric bed, the officer in charge of local authority residential accommodation would assess the same person as much too confused for its care. In one case the health authority dumped an old woman back in her home without any support in order to force the social services to take over her care. Certainly the reasons why confused older people became the responsibility of either the psychogeriatric department and therefore visited by a community psychiatric nurse (CPN) or visited by a social worker and under the wing of the social services department were hard to determine. Similarly the roles of CPNs and social workers were hard to differentiate.

The financial implications for the older person could be unfortunate. While hospital care remains free, most local authority-provided services are means tested. In my research this was most apparent in relation to respite care and day care. Two weeks in a psychogeriatric ward to give a husband or wife a rest could be free, whereas the same respite provided through an old people's home could cost around a £150 a week. Similarly many old people resent paying for lunch and transport to a local authority or voluntarily run day centre when the same day spent in a hospital day centre, which probably would have more facilities is free. A cynical reading of the motivation behind the Community Care Act would see it as a way of ironing out those anomalies by removing much of the care which is free to the client. There has been a steady erosion of free health services, many of which are vital to older people, for instance the services of opticians, dentists, chiropodists and hearing clinics. If these preventative services become more expensive or means tested then this valuable preventative aspect will be lost with a subsequent deterioration in the health and well-being of older people. Many may find that they can no longer afford new spectacles, well fitting dentures, effective hearing aids or regular chiropody which preserves mobility.

The NHS and Community Care Act, although gaining royal assent in June 1990, was not implemented until August 1993. Therefore at the time of writing it is not possible to discern its effects on the health and well-being of older people. What does it promise?

The rhetoric of the Act is 'choice' and 'consumerism'. Walker has set out four key characteristics:

- services that respond flexibly and sensitively to the needs of individuals and their carers;
- services that intervene no more than is necessary to foster independence;
- services that allow a range of options for consumers;
- services that concentrate on those with the greatest needs.

(Walker 1993)

Walker goes on to describe how the Act defines 'choice': 'giving people a greater individual say in how they live their lives and the services they need to help them'. (Walker 1993: 216). This choice is to be achieved by a process of care management where an individual and his/her needs are assessed in participation with a care manager. The services to meet these needs will be provided by a wide range of non-statutory providers. The role of the local authority is no longer to be the primary provider of services but the purchaser of care. It is responsible for assessing need, and managing the delivery of services but will only have a residual role in the actual provision of those services.

Although the Act is too new to make any assessment, policy analysts have been trying to tease out the possible implications. Walker has pointed out that the main thrust of the Act has been 'management-oriented rather than user-oriented' (1993: 218) and that its main concerns are cost rather than quality of care. He is therefore sceptical about its ability to enhance users' choices or increase participation in the assessment of need; this concern is also shared by Hoyes and Means who ask:

> To what extent is the consumer able to choose what he or she actually wants and to what extent is service access dependent upon the assessment and negotiation skills of a professional? How much choice does the client of a care manager have? Can they choose their care manager? Will there be enough independent providers to provide an adequate range of choice in all cases?
>
> (1993: 293)

Hoyes and Means are also concerned with the emphasis in the Act on the creation of markets in social care work and question whether this is the way to improve equity in social care and provide for those in greatest need, the fourth key characteristic of the new Act. They argue that conventional markets have a potential to create inequalities and that the 'quasi-markets' proposed in the Act could have similar effects:

> Will residential care providers compete for healthy elderly people, while ignoring those suffering from dementia and incontinence? Will the poor – constrained by lack of resources – be particularly disadvantaged?
>
> (Hoyes and Means 1993: 293)

Many of the anxieties surrounding the implementation of the NHS and Community Care Act are to do with a perceived lack of funding. Without adequate funding there are fears that services and benefits will increasingly be subjected to means testing and the burdens of social care will fall on already overstretched informal carers. This is a point taken up by Walker who questions the assumption that families can, will and should care for dependent older people. He warns that:

> research has shown that this confidence in familism is sometimes misplaced: family care can be both the best and the worst form of support (Qureshi and Walker 1989). If policy-makers continue to assume that it is always the soundest basis for care they will overlook inherent conflicts in the caring relationship and be guilty of imposing some destructive relationships on both carers and cared-for.
>
> (Walker 1993: 220)

The issue of informal care is a complex and contentious one and it is one to which we will return in Chapter 8 in considering the issue of social support.

Table 7.1 Estimated programme budget for health care services in England, 1986–87.

Programme	£ million	% of total on aged 65+
Acute in-patients	3519.2	45.8
Acute out-patients	1134.5	19.1
Obstetric in-patients	431.9	–
Obstetric out-patients	81.3	–
Geriatric in-patients	902.4	97.6
Young disabled	23.0	1
Geriatric out-patients	8.1	100
Mental handicap in-/out-patients	496.6	16.2
Mental illness in-patients	998.2	57
Mental illness out-patients	71.4	57
Non-psychiatric day patients	66.8	76.1
Psychiatric day patients	79.6	57
Other hospital	633.8	34.8
Health visiting	164.3	9.9
District nursing	331.6	74.6
Chiropody	34.5	89.7
Other community	4328.2	46.2
Total	10317.2	48.4

Source: Bosanquet and Gray (1989), Tables 26 and 28

Fears of underfunding of community care services are linked to diminishing resources in the hospital sector with anxieties that the closure of hospital beds before the resources become available in the community will represent a net loss of services. Any erosion of either hospital or community care services is likely to effect the health and wellbeing of older people as they are heavy users of the services of both as Table 7.1 shows.

Table 7.2 NHS estimated annual expenditure per head by age group in England, 1986–87

Age group	Expenditure per head (£)	% total expenditure
All births	1184.0	7.3
0–4	196.6	5.7
5–15	97.2	6.3
16–44	83.2	16.4
45–64	160.5	16.1
65–74	414.8	17.0
75–84	926.9	22.6
85+	1452.3	8.6

Source: Bosanquet and Gray 1989, Tables 27 and 28

The use older people make of the health services

Nearly half of all NHS expenditure goes on those over 65. Table 7.1 gives a breakdown of this expenditure with the percentage spent on those over 65. As well as the specialist geriatric services, those over 65 take up nearly half of the acute patient budget and about two-thirds of the community services. If we look at the per capita expenditure by age then it is clear that we consume more health care at birth and in old age, especially in extreme old age (see Table 7.2).

We are constantly bombarded with such phrases as the 'burden of dependency of older people' or talk of older people 'swamping' the health services which implies that older people are having more than their fair share of the health budget and depriving younger people of services which would benefit them more. Yet the figures to a large extent reflect the fact that both birth and death and the events leading up to death, which may span a few years, consume a lot of health service resources and nowadays most people do their dying in old age. It might prove a salutary exercise if we could do the sums in different ways and look at what people have consumed over a lifetime. If the expenditure per head of the 85 year olds could be averaged over their lifetime then we may get a very different picture of the share out of health resources.

The links between mortality and expenditure can be most clearly seen in the figures for hospital in-patient admissions as Christina Victor (1991: 114) has noted: 'The percentage of the population reporting a hospital in-patient stay shows a J-shaped distribution very similar to the pattern for mortality'. This can be seen in the bar diagram in Figure 7.1. (The kink in the curve for women between 16 and 44 can be accounted for by admissions for childbirth.)

Clearly the link to mortality is an oversimplification of the whole picture of spending on health. Hospitals also provide life-enhancing treatments as well as

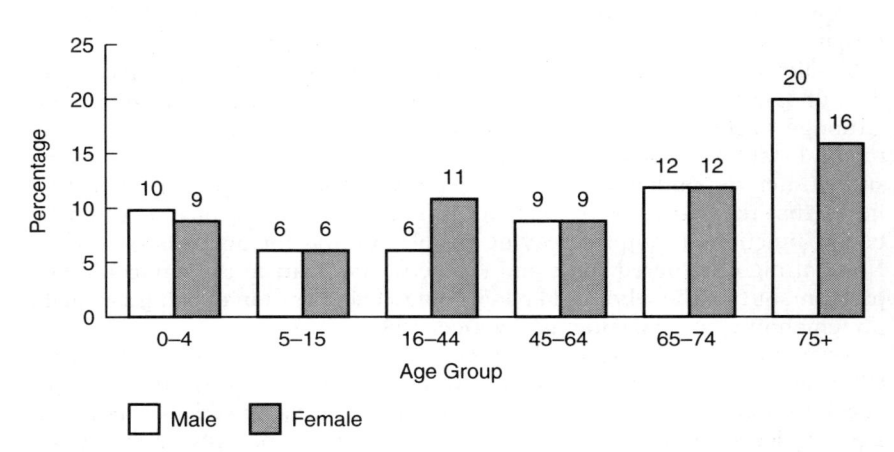

Figure 7.1 In-patient admissions in previous 12 months in Great Britain, 1987
Source: OPCS, 1988.

Table 7.3 Levels of satisfaction with the NHS (per cent) in Great Britain, 1987

	NHS as a whole		In-patients		Out-patients	
	Satisfied	Dissatisfied	Satisfied	Dissatisfied	Satisfied	Dissatisfied
65–74	45	30	78	6	70	7
75+	56	20	72	5	70	6
All ages	40	40	67	13	54	13

Per cent who thought there was need for improvement in the hospital services

	65–74	75+	All
Waiting time for elective surgery	80	77	87
Waiting time for out-patient appointments	74	69	83
Staffing by nurses in hospitals	65	49	75
Staffing by doctors in hospitals	64	47	70
Quality of hospital treatment	23	12	30
Quality of hospital nursing	15	7	21

Source: Bosanquet and Gray (1989), Tables 17 and 18

life saving ones. Nevertheless it is safe to say that the NHS is still very much an illness service and a great deal of effort goes into preventing and dealing with death. The issue of resource allocation within the NHS is a complicated one and one which has received a great deal of attention recently with the attempt to redress the balance between expenditure on hospitals and community care, and to find ways of rationing the services. This raises important ethical issues which we will address in the final chapter.

If older people are heavy users of the health services, are they satisfied with the service they receive? Levels of satisfaction expressed in large sample surveys is high as Table 7.3 shows. The only concerns were with waiting times for appointments and elective surgery and some concerns with the levels of hospital staff.

Smaller scale qualitative studies such as Wenger's (1988) also noted a good deal of satisfaction among those who had experienced hospital treatment, although again there was concern over the level of information given by medical staff. Nursing staff were always highly praised but, as in the sample survey, her respondents were concerned with the shortage of nurses. They noted that the nurses were 'rushed off their feet' and too busy to attend to bodily functions promptly, leaving people waiting for bedpans or washes. Noise at night bothered some and the very early start to the day could be a problem, but on the whole 'old people give the impression of being satisfied if undemanding hospital patients' (Wenger 1988: 49).

An area where older people do express complaint, and it is one which many GPs share, is the manner of discharge from hospital and the arrangements for adequate follow up care. Wenger reported people being sent home at very short notice without checking if carers were able to cope. GPs sometimes did not receive information about drugs and treatment and in some cases were not even informed of the discharge.

Health care and the management of health 121

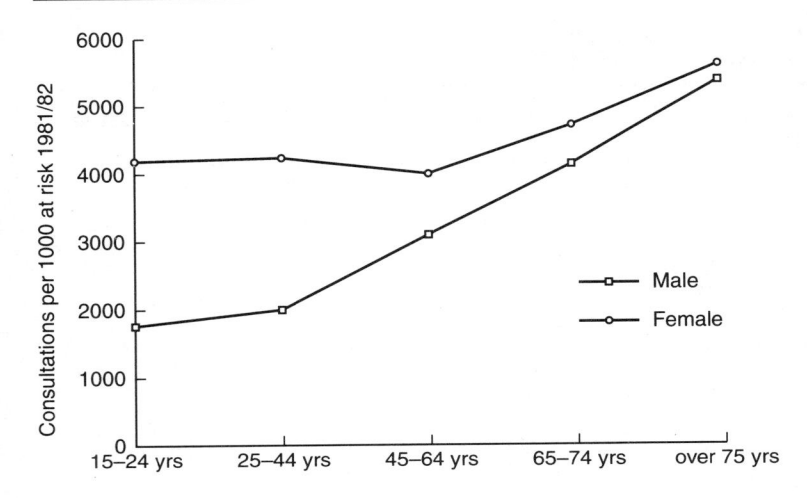

Figure 7.2 Consultations with GPs
Source: Royal College of General Practitioners, 1986

Use of General Practitioners

The service which is most frequently used and which is often the first point of contact is the General Practitioner service. This service is vital to older people but, it is one which is the least universally satisfying. Older people depend on their GP a great deal. The consultation rates (see Figure 7.2) show the proportions of older people who use the service. These data come from the Third National Morbidity survey of General Practitioners carried out by the Royal College of General Practitioners in 1982 (RCGP 1986). Unfortunately the data is not available for secondary analysis but we can discover gender differences and differences between age groups.

There are marked differences between men and women until the age of 65 but then the gap narrows with consultations increasing for both men and women. But these figures do not tell us whether a lot of men or women consult a little, or a few men or women consult a lot. It has been suggested that a small proportion of the older population use a great deal of the provision (Roos and Shapiro 1981). Is it the case that a small proportion of older people are consulting many times a year? Table 7.4 shows how frequently people consulted their GP during the year.

Around 30 per cent of those between 65 and 74 years and over a quarter of those over 75 years did not consult their GP at all. Twenty-seven per cent of men and 30 per cent of women between the ages 65 and 74 consulted their GP more than five times in the year. The figures are slightly higher for those over 75, 32 per cent for men and 35 per cent for women. The rest consulted between one and five times in the year. Can we identify any particular socioeconomic groups within the older population who consult their GP more than others? Secondary analysis of the GHS data allows for analysis of the consultations made to doctors in the two weeks prior to the survey along certain socioeconomic variables (see Table 7.5).

Table 7.4 Patients consulting per cent of persons present for the whole of the study year (age groups by frequency of consultation)

Frequency of consultation		All Ages	Age 65–74 years	Age 75 yrs and over
0	M	38	31	28.5
	F	28	28	25
1	M	17	13	11
	F	14	12	11
2–4	M	26	25	24
	F	28	25	24
5–9	M	10	15.5	16.5
	F	14	17	18
10–14	M	4	7	9
	F	7	8	9
15–29	M	2	4	6
	F	4	5	7
Over 30	M	0.1	0.4	1
	F	0.3	0.6	1.3

Source: Royal College of General Practitioners 1986.

The differences are predictable: women consult more than men, very old more than young-old, widowed more than single or married, working class more than middle class, council house tenants more than owner occupiers and those with a long standing illness or disability more than those without. Ebrahim and Hillier (1991) reviewing the use by Asian and Afro-Caribbean elders found that Asian elders were high users of GP services but low users of social services whereas Afro-Caribbean elders' use of health and social services was similar to the indigenous population. They maintain that the levels of GP consultation reflects the levels of morbidity and counter any suggestion that ethnic elders use the services inappropriately. In fact the consultation patterns reflect the patterns of morbidity in the older population as a whole and on that basis would seem to be at an appropriate level.

The issue of whether older people under or over consult is one which received a good deal of attention in the 1960s and 1970s (Williamson et al. 1964; Moen 1978; Tulloch and Moore 1979). Ford and Taylor (1985: 246), reviewing this evidence, concluded that 'we are unable to confirm the widely held view of the elderly as underconsulters'. Neither is there any evidence to show that older people are swamping the GPs' service with unnecessary consultations. The older women in Blaxter and Paterson's generational study (1982) were less likely to use the medical services than the younger ones because they felt they ought to use the service sparingly. Most of the older women in my study echoed the views of Blaxter and Paterson's cohort of older women. The overwhelming impression was that one should not bother the doctor unless absolutely necessary. This almost amounted to a moral code and relates to the moral imperative of not giving in to illness discussed in Chapter 2. Typical was one woman of 79, who said:

Table 7.5 Percentage who had consulted their doctor in the two weeks before the interviews

	Women % (n = 2090)	Men % (n = 1436)
All	19	17.5
Age groups		
65–74 years	17.5	16
Over 75 years	21	20
Marital status		
Married	16.5	17
Single	19.5	13.5
Widowed	21	20
Social class		
Non manual	17.5	15
Manual	20.5	20.5
Housing classes		
Rents from local authority	20.54	22.5
Owner occupier	18	15
Other rental	17.5	14.5
Education		
Some qualifications	14.5	11
No qualifications	15.5	18.5

Source: GHS 1985. Own analysis of unpublished data

> I always put it off – I say, it will go, or I can cope with it, and put it off until suddenly I say, you bloody fool, you'd better go and see him. I don't like going to doctors, I don't like the whole experience.

Others, like Mrs Barnard, in Chapter 5, were afraid of hearing something they did not want to hear. Yet others, like Sarah, went for regular check ups as a preventative measure. There was no evidence that older people visited their doctors inappropriately. The degree of help and satisfaction they receive is another matter.

Satisfaction with General Practitioners

Older people express a lot of satisfaction with the GP service in response to large sample surveys such as the British Social attitudes survey. But small scale qualitative studies such as Clare Wenger's study in rural Wales (1988) and my own (Sidell 1991) reveal issues which give cause for concern and which are not picked up in the more 'public' surveys. Wenger distinguished three such areas of concern: inadequate visiting, insensitivity and not giving as much information as needed or wanted. Many of her respondents, like Lily in Chapter

5, felt that the doctors were reluctant to visit them at home even when requested. As Wenger notes:

> Given the reluctance of elderly patients to 'trouble' the doctor, when attempts are made to establish contact it would seem that these should be taken as indicative of a high level of concern.
>
> (1988: 41)

Others in Wenger's study and their carers expressed the wish that the doctor would 'pop in' to give them reassurance or monitor change. However much this may seem an unrealistic expectation in today's highly pressurized system it is something which many feel would be of value to them.

Whilst acknowledging that many doctors are considered to be extremely kind and caring, older people and their carers can be particularly upset by the odd abrupt or insensitive remark made by some doctors who are often oblivious to this upset. Typical was Jim Wilson's GP who took a 'hearty' approach to prostate troubles. But as Wenger observes:

> While the professional moves on to the rest of a busy day, the old person in ill-health is more often than not left alone to mull over and weigh every remembered word of the exchange.
>
> (1988: 42)

The lack of information given to older people was a problem also for the respondents in my own study. Concern was expressed both with the giving and receiving of information. Many expressed the opinion that their point of view was not being taken seriously and they were not listened to. They felt that their GP was too busy either to listen to them or to explain things to them. In fact the unequal power relationship inherent in the doctor/patient relationship is difficult for younger, as well as older, people to negotiate. Older people rarely feel able to question or criticize their GP:

> the general impression gained of the relationship between doctor and old person is one of deference and social distance on the part of the patient, resulting in reluctance to ask questions, query treatment or report side-effects or lack of relief.
>
> (Wenger 1988: 43)

Helman (1990) believes that there is an almost inevitable 'culture clash' between doctors and their patients. This he argues is due to both differences in social class, economic status, legal status, gender and ethnic and religious background and to what he sees as a medical subculture. This subculture is inculcated into doctors through medical schools and hospitals and is based on the principles of scientific rationality and emphasis on objective measures and a dualistic approach to 'mind' and 'body'. Frustrating and irritating interactions between doctors and their older patients can result, particularly for those who also have a different ethnic background. This issue is discussed fully in Kenneth Blakemore and Maureen Boneham's book in this series (1993); they write:

> Being a patient and receiving medical attention not only involves following specialist advice or being expected to cooperate in being 'worked upon' by practitioners. The patient role also involves learning rules of

expected patient behaviour: for example, patients are usually expected to be rational and to explain their symptoms in an appropriate manner, to show pain in appropriate ways, and to comply with medical advice about diet, the therapies being administered, and so on. Medicine may therefore be seen as a social process, involving social rules, values and a culture; it is not simply a set of technical or scientific processes.

(Blakemore and Boneham 1993: 104–105)

If the GP's surgery is a subculture with different expectations of behaviour from that of many of its patients then perhaps it is that which should be viewed as 'exotic and awkward' rather than the patients (Blakemore and Boneham 1993). But it is the unequal power relationship that invests control of the situation in the doctors which therefore allows them to set the social rules and norms of behaviour that may put many of the patients at a disadvantage. If doctors, as most of them do, genuinely want to help their patients, then some breaking down of these cultural barriers is necessary. Blakemore and Bonham suggest that attention is needed to key 'problem areas' such as language, providing enough information and explanation in an accessible form, understanding nutritional traditions and requirements of different cultures, and a sensitivity to gender issues, especially in relation to Asian communities. Perhaps more importantly the issue of racism in the health service is cause for great concern. They discuss different levels of racism, direct, organizational and institutional which affect not so much a person's access to medical care but to his or her access to satisfactory care (Ferraro 1987). They may also encounter ageism manifested by the 'what can you expect at your age' attitude which has been the experience of many older people, black and white (Sidell 1992). If older people are disappointed in their encounters with their doctors and find them less than satisfactory, then as well as the problems of gaining equitable treatment, there will be other consequences. For instance they may be less likely to comply with treatment. This can happen with drug therapies in which the effects and possible side-effects are not sufficiently well explained.

Both Wenger's respondents and the older women in my study were concerned about the drugs that they were prescribed. Like Mrs Gerrard, they felt that they were taking too many, the drugs were not doing them any good and that sometimes they felt they were positively harmful. Many like Mrs Gerrard did not question the doctor and went on taking them until another doctor took over their care. Others simply did not take the medicines prescribed but neither did they tell the doctor and so could be put at risk if the drugs were potentially life saving. Burns and Phillipson point out some disturbing features of the drug-based therapy given to older people:

- In 1982 older people in the United Kingdom received 15.9 prescriptions per head compared to 5.2 younger people and they are taken for longer periods.
- Repeat prescriptions without consultations are common and are often made out by ancillary staff.
- Older people take a lot of over-the-counter medication and the interaction with prescribed medications is rarely monitored.

- Most drugs are safety tested on younger people and the possible harmful effects on older people are not understood.

While acknowledging that many drugs are life saving and of immense benefit to older people Burns and Phillipson caution that:

> The elderly are two or three times more likely to suffer harm from medicines than younger people (George 1981), and the mortality from this form of iatrogenic disease rises exponentially with age.
>
> (Burns and Phillipson 1988: 199)

The high level of 'accidents, injury and poisoning' found in older people and discussed in Chapter 3 was related to the use of prescribed medicines.

The problem for the GP lies in the nature of the health problems presented by older people. The highly symptomatic but 'incurable' illnesses which many bring to their GP presents them with a dilemma. They have little in their armoury with which to deal with these conditions. When faced with an old person seeking relief from the chronic pain of arthritis or anxiety and depression caused by loneliness or bereavement they have only painkillers, anti-inflammatory or psychotophic drugs to offer. The skills of physiotherapists and occupational therapists which potentially could help with mobility and flexibility problems are not widely available outside of hospitals. Counselling, which might help relieve emotional pain, is mainly provided by voluntary agencies such as the bereavement counselling agency, CRUSE. Easing therapies such as massage and acupuncture, have not generally been available on the NHS. This could change in practices where GPs become fundholders. They could buy in a whole range of therapies and provide a very different type of service to their patients. However the whole range of non-orthodox medicine has developed independently and with a degree of mutual hostility.

Alternative or complementary therapies

As we discussed in Chapter 1, alternative or complementary therapies which include a wide and varied range of treatments such as acupuncture, homeopathy, naturopathy, osteopathy, chiropractics, aromatherapy, reflexology and herbalism take a much more 'holistic' view of health (Aakster 1986). Mind, body and soul are indivisible and health is a matter of balance, harmony and equilibrium with the immediate and wider social and physical environment. Enthusiasts for these therapies suggest that they have a lot to offer older people affected by chronic conditions such as cardiovascular ailments, strokes and arthritis. (Scrutton 1992). Yet exponents of western medicine remain deeply sceptical about the benefits to be had from alternative therapies and want proof of their efficacy before endorsing their use, but as we noted in Chapter 1, alternative therapies do not operate within a scientific paradigm and resent being judged by these standards. Many therapies operate with different expectations. They may not be seeking 'cures' but attempting to bring relief from symptoms which is very much what many older people are seeking when they consult with their doctors. Research on users of alternative medicine suggests that most sought help because of the failure of biomedicine to effect a cure or because they were dissatisfied with their doctor. What they valued most was the 'holistic' approach which considered the 'personal context of illness' and they liked the more equal and informed relationship with their therapist (Sharma 1990).

Although alternative therapies are sometimes known as complementary, there are very few examples where allopathic and complementary therapies truly complement each other in the British system. This approach is much more common in other parts of Europe where the distinction between orthodox and non-orthodox medicine is less rigidly drawn. In France and Germany for example both are available under the standard health insurance schemes (Ooijendijk et al. 1981), and the European Community is seeking to regulate the practice and training of practitioners in non-orthodox therapies which would help allay the anxieties which arise from the uncontrolled proliferation of these practices (Lewith and Aldridge 1991).

There are some attempts to integrate orthodox and non-orthodox medicine, for instance the Marylebone centre in London. This is an NHS health centre run by Dr Patrick Pietroni where NHS doctors work in conjunction with a range of complementary therapists providing acupuncture, massage, osteopathy and healing to all its patients free of charge. Another very strong advocate of complementary therapies is Helen Passant, a sister on what used to be an old style 'geriatric' ward at the Churchill Hospital in Oxford. She has learned many of the skills of non-orthodox therapies, and in turn trained other nurses in aromatherapy, massage and herbalism and she explores a wide range of diets and healing therapies in her efforts to improve the health and well-being of her patients. Here she describes her work:

> I began to look outside conventional methods of care – at complementary therapies which would enhance our nursing. . . . I began to massage my patients, using herbal oils, and taught my staff to do likewise. . . . We also began to use essential oils to enhance the effect of massage and discovered that we were able to reduce conventional sedative drugs to a minimum. . . . We used the oils intuitively. Lavender and rose geranium were used for patients suffering from dementia; cedarwood for mood swings and chest problems; cardamom for memory; lavender for headache and muscular pain.
>
> (Passant 1990: 27)

In the main it is only those who are able to pay who can choose non-orthodox therapies, but many older people use herbal remedies and have a whole repertoire of self-care therapies, particularly for such conditions as arthritis where the doctor's medicine is of little help.

Self-health care

In the maintenance of health and well-being personal health care has probably more day to day significance than formal medical care (Hickey 1986). Yet as Kathryn Dean has argued, 'little is known about either the range of self-care behaviour or the combination of factors and processes determining its development' (1986: 60). She defines self-care in the following way:

> Self-care involves the range of activities individuals undertake to enhance health, prevent disease, evaluate symptoms and restore health. These activities are undertaken by lay people on their own behalf, either separately or in participation with professionals. Self-care includes decisions to do nothing, self-determined actions to promote health or treat illness, and decisions to seek advice in lay, professional and alternative care networks, as well as evaluation of and decisions regarding action based on that advice.
>
> (Dean 1986: 62)

She stresses the importance of a decision to do nothing, to 'let nature take its course' and also the interaction of self care and professional care. She believes that the two should not be seen as dichotomous. The decision to seek professional care is part of an individual's self-care behaviour and so is the decision to comply or not to comply with professionally prescribed treatment. Ideally all of these decisions should be based on basic health knowledge and skills but Kathryn Dean has shown that this is often lacking among older people (Dean 1982). Five components of such knowledge have been identified in a review of self-health care and older people, carried out for the World Health Organization (Coppard et al. 1984). These are:

- simple diagnostic skills – which the individual might use to estimate her or his health status, e.g. breast self-examination, monitoring pulse rate, checking temperature;
- skills relevant to simple acute conditions – including treatment of the common cold and everyday illnesses, and first-aid for non life-threatening conditions;
- skills needed to treat chronic illness – such as self-monitoring and following prescribed regimes;
- skills for disease prevention and health promotion – including exercise, diet, avoiding tobacco and alcohol abuse, good dental hygiene and healthy lifestyles;
- health information skills – such as what steps to take prior to seeking professional treatment, how to obtain health information and how to gain access to formal care.

There have been encouraging developments in improving the self-health care skills and knowledge of older people but these are patchy and left to community and voluntary groups. One of the best examples has been the work of the Beth Johnson Foundation in Stoke-on-Trent which has pioneered a variety of methods such as health courses and talks, activities and exercise, accessible health information and advice as well as a scheme of peer health counselling (Bernard and Ivers, 1986; Bernard, 1988,1989). We will return to this issue of health education for older people in the last chapter as we look to the future.

Self-help groups are a potential source of both education and support for older people (Bernard 1985, 1988). They tend to centre round a particular condition, such as the Alzheimer's Disease Society and perform other functions than education and support. They act as a lobby for better research and resources and sometimes become involved in the provision of services. Gareth Williams claims that self-help is 'Janus-faced' (1989: 138) and straddles the two ideologies of individualism and collectivism:

> in one guise it celebrates individual freedom against a corporatist state, however illusory or limited this freedom may be in practice; in the other it articulates a collective defence of communal resources, however paltry and dehumanising these may be in reality.
>
> (ibid)

The belief that self help groups represent the 'twin virtues of self-reliance and reciprocity' (Richardson and Goodman 1983: 1) ignores the tension inherent in this uneasy relationship between two opposing ideologies. In practice Williams believes that self-help groups tend to fall into those which are inner directed and focus more on self-care and individualism and those which are outer directed and overtly political. But he believes that invariably individualism becomes the dominant partner, reinforcing an emphasis on individual responsibility for health. Moreover there is a danger that:

> self-help groups, and other voluntary associations, provide governments who are so inclined with a ready excuse for dismantling the statutory health services.
>
> (Williams 1989: 155)

This theme of individual and collective responsibility for health will be developed further in the next two chapters when we consider personal resources for health and social support and the future prospects for health in old age.

8

Personal resources and social support

Introduction

The diversity of health experience amongst those designated 'elderly' is clear whether we take statistical data or individual accounts as evidence. Age is part, but only a part, of the picture. Most people die in old age and there is a greater risk of chronic illness and disability with increased age. Gender is also important, as we saw in Chapter 3, men on average die at younger ages than women but women suffer more symptomatic but non-life threatening conditions. The evidence for differences based on ethnicity is more difficult to discern partly because of a lack of data but partly because it is difficult to disentangle from the effects of socioeconomic disadvantage (Norman 1985; Blakemore and Boneham 1993). The links between poor health and socioeconomic disadvantage throughout the life span have been forcibly made (Townsend and Davidson 1986; Whitehead 1987; Arber and Ginn 1991a and b), emphasizing the cumulative effects on people as they age. Lifestyles have come under scrutiny with a number of 'habits' identified as harmful to health such as smoking, excessive alcohol consumption, lack of exercise and poor diet. But to confound the picture even more there are plenty of examples of very old men and women who have lived materially impoverished lives, never exercised, been nourished on dripping 'butties', even been heavy smokers, who are hale and hearty at 80 or 90. Clearly there are other dimensions. Constitution, personality and social supports are other candidates for filling in the gaps in the picture of what makes for health in old age. Work in the field of genetics indicates that we are programmed to withstand or succumb to certain diseases, but still there seems to be another dimension which has particularly exercised the minds of psychologists – that of personality, some difficult to define 'characteristic' of a person, developed through the life span, which not only seems to buffer them against diseases but also comes to their aid if illness does take hold.

Health in old age is a complex mixture of biology and biography and this chapter seeks to explore these dimensions. However I will not try to identify which factors most influence a person's health chances but instead explore the range of resources available to older people both to withstand disease and to cope with ill-health and move towards the health end of Antonovsky's health-ease-dis-ease continuum.

Threats to health have been described as stressors (Antonovsky 1979, 1987) and these can be microbiological, such as harmful bacteria or viruses, or sociocultural experiences. A great deal of work has been done which attempts to link stressful life events to certain diseases including heart disease, musculo-skeletal conditions and depression (Holmes and Rahe 1967; Dohrenwend and Dohrenwend 1974; Paykel 1974; Brown and Harris 1978). Although correlations are found between certain life events and disease these are by no means universal and the question always comes back to why one person becomes depressed or develops heart disease in response to a stressful life and another with an equally stressful record does not. Attention has shifted from identifying the stressful events to looking at the way people cope with such events. Antonovsky proposes that:

> Confronting a stressor results in a state of tension, with which one must deal. Whether the outcome will be pathological, neutral, or salutary depends on the adequacy of tension management.
>
> (1987: xii)

This 'tension management' in turn depends on the adequacy of certain resistance resources and these have been identified as constitutional strength, social support, material resources and personality dispositions (Lazarus and Launier 1978; Pearlin and Schooler, 1978; Kobasa *et al.* 1981). The chapter will begin by addressing the issue of constitutional strength and then go on to explore the impact of material resources in countering and mitigating the effects of ill-health. Social support which has been identified as a vital source of help to people as they age, will be discussed in relation to issues of dependency and interdependency. The more individual resource of personality will be explored in relation to both the ways people cope with stressors and to the actions that people take for health.

The notion of resources for health highlights questions about responsibility for health which were raised in Chapter 2 in relation to people's beliefs and attitudes to health. In this chapter we will explore individualism and collectivism as ideological imperatives for determining where responsibility lies for health and the care of dependent individuals.

A strong constitution

We talk of being 'blessed' with a strong constitution, it is something we are born with. Thomas Whiteside and Miss Hamish could be said to have a strong constitution although biologically we have no way of knowing and Sarah thought that she was strong in spite of her arthritis. Laura also saw herself as physically strong and young for her years and Kate, in spite of neglecting herself, was physically fit. Mrs Gerrard and Mrs Barnard on the other hand, both saw themselves as constitutionally weak and neither did Lily think she was physically robust. The idea of strength and weakness to withstand disease was one much used in the lay concepts of disease causation discussed in Chapter 2. Much of this contitutional resource people think of as familial – a matter of heredity.

Modern genetic research indicates that our susceptibility to certain diseases and our potential life-span is programmed. Hayflick's work on cellular tissue points to the existence of a biological clock ticking away at a pre-programmed rate (Coni et al. 1992), but the clock can be upset by unprogrammed events. DNA, the carrier of genetic information, is susceptible to damage by internal and external agents such as heat, cold, ultraviolet light, irradiation and free oxygen (superoxide) radicals causing alterations in the information they carry. Coni et al. explain:

> These alterations, called mutations, occur particularly as a result of irradiation and other harmful stimuli, but can also occur on a spontaneous basis. Mutations fundamentally affect the DNA and thus the encoded information, and this is one of the mechanisms whereby environmental factors influence the integrity of the cell, the tissue, and thus the organism.
>
> (1992: 50)

The body has various mechanisms for detecting, repairing or eliminating these alterations which threaten the homeostasis of the organism. One such stress resisting resource is thought to be the immunopotentiating and immunosuppressing mechanisms which the body has as a form of defence. The efficiency of this system has a tendency to decline in old age and thus increases the risk of disease. The overall capacity to maintain homeostasis seems to be impaired in extreme old age. The maintenance of bodily temperature is a prime example of this. In frail older people body temperature is put at risk in extremes of external temperatures, resulting in hypothermia. This is a good example of biological factors reacting with environmental and social factors to cause bodily harm. Having a strong constitution is clearly a bonus but it may not be enough to counteract the negative effects of poverty and social disadvantage.

Material resources

Inequalities in health measured by mortality, morbidity and self assessment show a strong relationship to social class and the related variables of income, housing and education. Poverty, poor housing and little education have a powerful negative influence on health (Victor 1991; Arber and Ginn 1993). As well as the statistical evidence on the impact of economic deprivation on health, the media frequently provide graphic accounts of malnutrition and hypothermia. None of the people depicted in the case studies were representative of the most materially disadvantaged older people in our society but the late David Widgery, a GP who practiced in the East End of London, provides harrowing evidence of the ravages of life at the bottom of the economic pile. He compares this with 'the affluent elderly' who he says:

> are in the prime of their life. Exactly as pictured in the pension adverts, they are enjoying the fruits of their lives, relishing the challenge of their gardens and the company of their grandchildren. But for the East End pensioner, the picture is often the reverse: poverty and isolation . . . Rather than old age being some universal state of being, it reflects quite precisely the class circumstances of the life that preceded it . . . Our duration of life and cause of death will be the end products of the inequalities in the use made of our bodies. And for surprising numbers of male manual workers, retirement after a hard working life, which was as physically demanding in their fifties as their twenties, is followed by premature death from preventable causes, from a stroke, lung cancer, or a heart attack. Perhaps more tragically still, an East End working life will often be followed, not by well-earned retirement but a non-fatal stroke or early dementia . . . which will render a once independent and active person chronically dependent.
>
> (Widgery 1991: 124, 125)

The notion that old age acts as a leveller in terms of material advantage and disadvantage has been shown not to be the case (Taylor and Ford 1983). Studies of economic disadvantage in Britain have shown that older people make up a large proportion of those in poverty, defined as living on or below the benefits level. But as Arber and Ginn (1993: 34) point out: 'there has been a tendency to conceive of elderly people as a homogeneous, "structurally dependent", group who are all disadvantaged by low income'. Arber and Ginn go on to argue, on the basis of their analysis of national data, that the income of older people in fact shows 'considerable differentiation', they are not 'universally poor' and they confirm David Widgery's evidence from practice that their present economic position reflects their previous position in the labour market and for women, their reproductive roles. Widows are particularly disadvantaged compared to men and never married women, with working class widows at the bottom of the economic scale and middle class older men at the top.

In Chapter 3 we saw how social class was related to the incidence of chronic illness and disability, that working-class older people had a higher incidence of chronic illness. Class is therefore a resistance resource in relation to chronic illness and disability. Arber and Ginn show that there is approximately a five-year class gap in disability. That women from Class V are more likely to be functionally disabled than women from the upper middle-class who are five years older and the picture is similar for men. They therefore argue that chronological age is less appropriate than class as a measure of chronic illness and disability.

Material resources have an immediate impact on health and well-being as well as cumulative effects. They can mitigate some of the unpleasant symptoms of chronic illness and disability, but conversely the lack of material resources can exacerbate the symptoms. Because of the difficulties of measuring social class of older people, especially older women, as an indicator of present material circumstances Arber and Ginn used three measures: income, whether

134 Resources for health

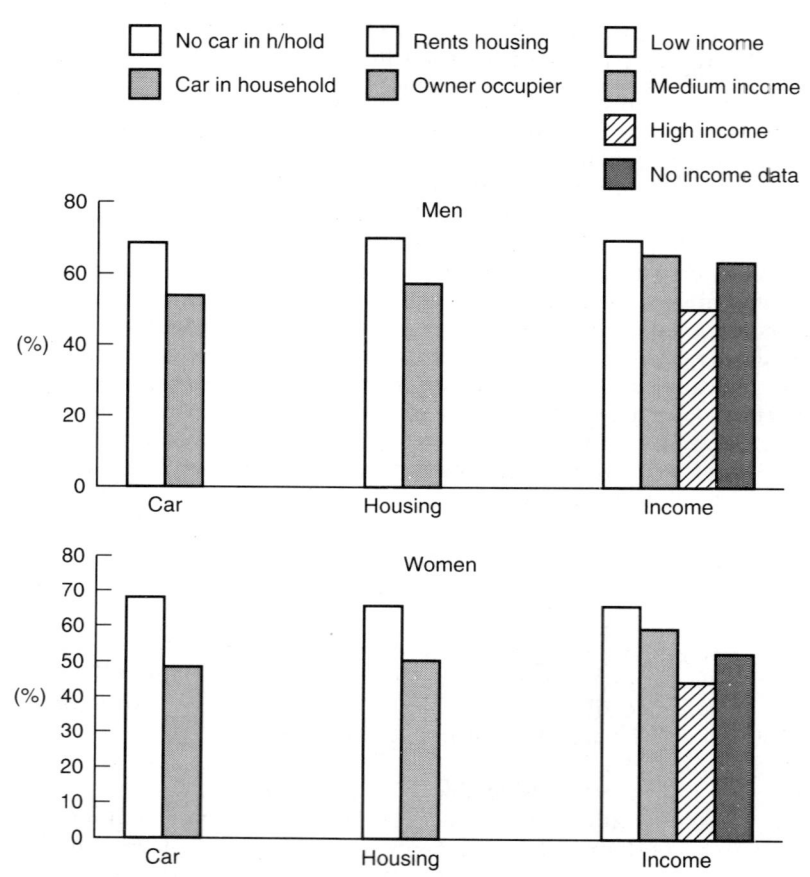

Figure 8.1 Self-assessed health: Percentage without good health, by access to material resources, elderly men and women.
Source: Arber and Ginn, 1993: 42.

the home is owned or rented, and whether there is a car in the household. Using data from the General Household Survey (GHS) they cross tabulated these variables with the self-assessment of health variable. The material circumstances of those older people who assessed their own health as poor is shown in Figure 8.1.

This table shows a clear link between low income, rented accommodation and having no car. They comment:

> These findings suggest that material advantage is critical for an elderly person's sense of well-being. This is likely to be because current material resources enable greater participation in desired leisure and social activities, and promote a sense of autonomy and independence. Although current material resources available to an elderly person are likely to

influence the experience of disability they do not affect its incidence. The latter represents the accumulated outcome of an elderly person's occupational and material position over the life course.

(Arber and Ginn 1993: 43)

Compensating for both material disadvantage and constitutional weakness manifested in ill-health has been a major policy aim of the welfare state since Beveridge. Titterton (1992) has described this as the 'old paradigm' of welfare to be contrasted with the 'new paradigm'. Fiona Williams, in a review of the arguments for a 'new paradigm of welfare' summarizes the criticisms of the 'old paradigm':

> individuals and their welfare needs have been understood passively within categories of researchers', providers' or policy-makers own making (socio-economic groups, children at risk, disabled, old etc). In so far as individuals' own needs and strategies have been studied, then such studies have tended towards a pathological view of poverty, ill-health and so on.
>
> (Williams, forthcoming)

Within this paradigm there is little scope for the 'creative human agent'. Williams identifies three distinct ways in which the new paradigm breaks with the old, by:

- providing an analytical framework for understanding the dialectical relationship between personal history and the social and material world;
- expanding the study of 'mediating structures' beyond formal welfare provision to include people's own psychological and social strategies;
- expanding the focus of study to include the resilience and resistance of 'the invulnerable'.

What are the implications of this new paradigm of welfare for older people? In the old paradigm older people constituted a high risk group, 'the elderly', regardless of whether the experience of individual older people warranted this categorization. Locating the individual's personal history within the social and material world and taking account of people's own psychology and social strategies acknowledges the diversity of older people's experience. Focusing on 'the invulnerables' amongst the older population provides a much more positive image of old age. Although there would be some gains in this shift in the paradigm of welfare, it is a shift which puts more emphasis on individualism and individual responsibility for health. The new paradigm of welfare is concerned with issues of personal coping and social support.

Personality resources for coping

A difficult to define characteristic of personality is thought to act as a 'buffering' reaction to stress (Lazarus 1966, Pearlin and Schooler 1978; Kobasa *et al.* 1981, 1982). Individuals cope with stressful life events by first appraising the event cognitively and then taking action to deal with the event. Kobasa *et al.* argue that personality dispositions influence this process. Personality dispositions affect the way the life event is perceived. Certain dispositions will encourage a more optimistic appraisal of the situation, perhaps taking a longer perspective or contextualizing the event so that it does not seem so bad. Personality dispositions will, in the light of how the event is perceived, activate an appropriate response. Kobasa *et al.* explain:

> What particular personality dispositions mitigate the otherwise debilitating effects of stressful life events? Specifically, they are those that have the cognitive appraisal effect of rendering the events as not so meaningless, overwhelming, and undesirable, after all, and the action effect of instigating coping activities that involve interacting with and thereby transforming the events into a less stressful form rather than avoiding them (Lazarus 1966). Persons with personality dispositions of this sort possess a valuable aid in avoiding illness-provoking biological states.
>
> (1982: 169)

Kobasa *et al.* (1982) formulated a concept of 'hardiness' which, they claim, functions as a stress resisting resource and so decreases the effect of stressful life events and the likelihood of resultant illness. Important elements of hardiness are commitment, control and challenge. Commitment represents a tendency to become involved in events or encounters rather than feeling alienated from them. Committed persons are more likely to try to understand an event and take action rather than avoiding the situation. This is linked to the control disposition of 'hardy' persons who are more likely to see themselves as being able to influence events rather than feeling helpless in the face of them. It represents the opposite of what Seligman termed 'learned helplessness' (1975). This sense of control leads to actions which are capable of transforming a stressful event into something which is less harmful. In terms of challenge, 'hardy' persons are those who relish change and see it as the norm. They see changes as 'interesting incentives to grow rather than threats to security' (Kobasa *et al.* 1982: 170).

Kobasa *et al.* go on to discuss how this personality disposition to 'hardiness' might interact with other resistance resources such as "constitution" or "social support"'. They suggest that 'hardy' personalities would be likely to engage in positive health practices such as exercise, good diet etc. which might mitigate a weak constitution or strengthen even more an already strong one. Another interaction which they suggest might be effective in preserving health would be the utilization of social support as 'hardy' persons would seek out and use support actively when faced with a stressful situation.

By the time people reach the last phase of the life cycle their 'hardiness' will have been put to the test many times. In discussing adjustment in later life Peter Coleman says: 'If old age has a special character in this regard it is the likelihood of unwanted changes occurring, sometimes also in close proximity and often unprepared for' (Coleman 1993: 98). He goes on to say that 'the capacity to adjust to life's changes does not appear to be diminished in later life, rather enhanced'. (ibid.: p98). Unfortunately little emphasis is given to how older people do adjust to potentially quite devastating life events such as loss of role, loss of a partner, sometimes accompanied by loss of a home and often loss of income. Much of the focus is on the minority who do not cope well with their losses. This is to be expected given that they will be the ones who seek help and so come to the attention of the health and welfare agencies, as well as giving cause for concern for relatives and friends. Identifying what it is that enables many older people to maintain equilibrium in the face of adversity may well be more fruitful than studying those who do not cope.

Elizabeth Colerick has identified a concept of 'stamina' in later life to describe the qualities that 'distinguish older persons who demonstrate emotional resilience despite age-related losses and life change' (Colerick 1985: 997). She includes 'mental vigour, vitality and endurance' as aspects of 'stamina'. She writes:

> High levels of stamina entail resilience and 'staying power': the strength (physical or moral) to withstand disease, fatigue or hardship. Although physical strength often wanes in later life, internal stamina reflects well-tested convictions that obstacles are surmountable and that personal growth is an outcome of personal struggle.
>
> (ibid.)

Her concept of 'stamina' has many similarities to Kobasa's 'hardiness' and like 'hardiness' people with 'stamina', it is argued, will be able to appraise a situation which threatens their well-being and move forward to feel 'challenged and self-confident' rather than helpless. Colerick suggests a model for current functioning in relation to stamina which is the result of 'adaptive potential' and 'cognitive appraisal', or 'personal outlook'.

The factors making up 'adaptive potential' relate to personal and social resources of earlier life, family origins and early childhood experiences, education and past health. The factors making up 'cognitive appraisal' or 'personal outlook' which is positive and likely to lead to 'stamina' develop over the years and are made up of two dimensions: one, the probability that the self will triumph over adversity – triumph meaning a sense of 'mastery' and control; and two, that the self is not isolated and can call on help in hard times. Colerick subjected the model to some complicated empirical testing on 68 older men and women and their identified significant others. Although she acknowledges that there are some methodological weaknesses in the study she does report some interesting findings:

- that older people with high 'stamina' have learned through the years that change is inevitable, challenging and manageable;
- that triumph perceptions in later life flow from years of success in acting on the environment;
- that older people with a triumphal outlook will look beyond age-related limitations for new ways to use energy – increasing understanding, extending skills, discovering more abilities;
- that educational attainment is by far the most powerful predictor of stamina in the later years;
- that advantaged childhood beginnings predict later life stamina, but only by increasing perceptions of support in late adulthood – there are no direct effect of family origins on current functioning.

One of the most important findings of her study is that educational attainment is the strongest predictor of stamina in later life. An equally important aspect, she suggests, is that it is:

> a testimony to the presence of earlier experience in later life. The boundaries of old age as a biological life stage are expanded to include a social and psychological past.
>
> (Colerick 1985: 1005)

The availability and use made of social support is also seen as a key factor in coping.

Social supports

A great deal of emphasis is given to the value of social support as a resource for maintaining health and well-being. Early work in the 1970s by Cassel (1976) an epidemiologist and Caplan (1974) a community physician in the USA and Brown and Harris (1978) in England focused on the 'protective' element in social support. Others have gone so far as to claim that it may directly influence mortality (Beckman and Syme 1979; Blazer 1982). Broadly there are two hypotheses relating to the effect of social support on health. One is that social support enhances health and well-being directly and intrinsically. The other is that social support acts as a buffer against the effects of stressful experiences — that it has an important effect in enabling people to cope with stressors.

The 'direct effect' hypothesis works in two ways. First there is the impact on self-esteem which is bolstered by feeling loved and liked and being able to reciprocate that love and affection. A secondary effect is provided by a sense of security that someone will be there to provide support in the event of distressing circumstances (Thoits 1982). The buffering effect is supposed to act by protecting people from the pathogenic effects of stress. Supported individuals can readily redefine the potential harm which threatens as well as having another resource at their disposal (Cohen and Wills 1985).

Before reviewing the evidence we have for the impact of social support on older people we need to unpick the term 'social support' which Hazel Qureshi (1990) has called a 'portmanteau' term. Who is it that provides social support and what is the nature of the support provided?

Social support is taken to be the support people give and take within their social relationships, usually understood to include family, friends and neighbours. The term normally excludes support from statutory workers. The term 'support' is vague and attempts have been made to break it down into more meaningful components. Vachon and Stylianos (1988) identified four such components when investigating the support available to bereaved people. These were:

- emotional or affective support,
- moral or appraisal support,
- informational support,
- instrumental or practical support.

Cohen and Wills (1985) reviewing the literature suggested a similar list: esteem support, informational support, social companionship and instrumental support. Weiss (1974), focusing on emotional support, broke down the concept into five functions: attachment and intimacy, social integration, nurturance, reassurance of worth and guidance.

Two basic characteristics seem to emerge from all this. One is about love, affection and affirmation. The other is a practical element, providing help and advice. Other distinctions have been made between crisis and everyday routine support (Veiel 1985) and between 'enacted' and 'perceived' support (Tardy 1985). The perceived availability of support would most likely relate to a crisis situation where an individual feels they can rely on someone if necessary although that person may not routinely be engaged in providing support. This latter can be very important to older people. Knowing that they can call on someone in an emergency can bring a comforting sense of security.

Whelan (1993: 87) has identified two approaches used in measures of social support:

1 Those looking at objective social conditions such as marital status, household composition, reported frequency of interaction with kin, friends and neighbours and membership of clubs and organizations.
2 Those relating to the functional content of relationships such as the degree to which they involve flows of affection, emotional concern or tangible aid.

As Whelan points out the first type, although indicating a level of social integration and participation, is really a measure of social contact. This is useful in identifying social isolation but evidence of social contact does not tell us anything about the value of those contacts, quantity does not guarantee quality. It is the second of Whelan's two types which is an attempt to measure the quality of the relationship. Qureshi (1990) has reviewed the various attempts to measure social support and relate it to health. She points out that the rationale for the first type of approach to measuring social support is that it indicates the potential support resource. Although there is no necessary connection between the number of social relationships and the quality of the support received, Qureshi cites a number of studies which have shown an association between the number of ties and health outcomes, but she goes on to comment: 'These *macro-level studies* provide little enlightenment as to how social support operates, and which aspects of it exactly are health protective, or in what degree' (Qureshi 1990: 40).

Micro-level studies using the second of Whelan's two approaches focus on the quality of relationships and have identified the health giving potential of the support provided by a 'confidante'. Lowenthal (1965) found a positive relationship between good health, high morale and the presence of a confidante among older people and more recent work by Elaine Murphy (1982) with older people in London has gone so far as to show that a confiding relationship is protective against depression.

Qureshi points out that the methodological problems associated with both measuring the input of social support and the health outcome, in terms of increased morale or the protective potential of the support, are legion. Methods vary, some use in-depth qualitative interviews and observation, others self completed questionnaires; there is a bewildering array of psychometric measures on offer. Nevertheless some common findings have emerged. Kessler et al. (1985) reviewed the evidence for the stress buffering effects of social support and indicate that emotional support provides a strong buffering role whereas a high level of social participation indicated by membership of affiliated networks did not. The evidence for instrumental support was unclear. Cohen and Wills (1985) in a similar review also found evidence for the buffering effects of emotional support and also that the integration/participation level was important for general well-being. These reviews are not age-specific and whilst the findings are relevant to all age groups there are special concerns about the availability and need for social support amongst older people.

Dorothy Jerrome (1981, 1991) has used qualitative research methods, in-depth interviews and observation to investigate the impact of friendship on the health of older people. Her work is in the best traditions of qualitative research, providing insight and understanding of a little researched area. She discusses three levels of support: the emotional, the cognitive and the instrumental. Jerrome says of friendship:

> It is an expression of individuality. The relationship is characterised by intimacy, dependability, mutual support and reciprocity . . . .The activities shared by friends include the provision of emotional support, reciprocal visiting, mutually enjoyable social activities and help with transport.
>
> (Jerrome 1990: 56)

She argues that at the cognitive level friends are important in establishing the norms of illness behaviour and in forming attitudes to health and illness. Achieving a balance between stoicism and self indulgence will all be negotiated between friends, resolving such dilemmas as whether to seek help from a doctor, whether to question medication, whether to take to one's bed:

> Members of the social network convey information, monitor performance, assess behaviour and make judgements. They provide guidelines for behaviour. Collectively they establish ways of coping with personal change.
>
> (Jerrome 1990: 52)

Being without friends and socially isolated makes it more difficult to cope with health crises, but Dorothy Jerrome accepts that 'friendship is not primarily instrumental'. This is not to imply that friends do not give practical help but this is usually based on the principle of reciprocity. Prolonged ill-health can upset the balance of reciprocity making friendships vulnerable to ill-health. She describes how friends sometimes attempt to suppress their symptoms in order to preserve a friendship. Where frailty and symptoms are unable to be hidden friends sometimes withdraw because of feelings of helplessness and a heightened sense of their own vulnerability. Often the withdrawal is mutual where sufferers lose confidence in their ability to fulfil the obligations of a friend. There are exceptions, however: 'There are also

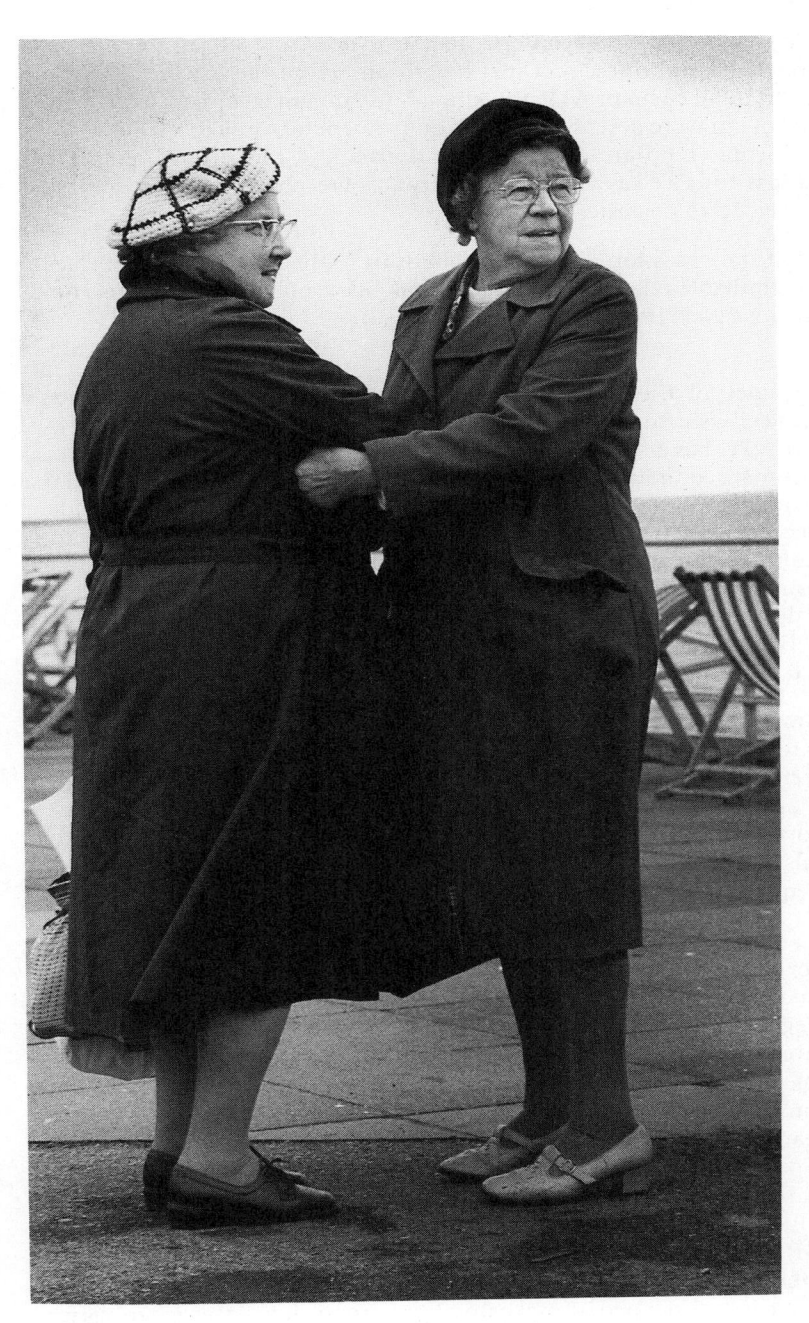

Friendship
Photograph: Georgina Ravenscroft

friendships which do not conform to the expectation of failure: frailty is accommodated and unreciprocated help is an acceptable feature'. (Jerrome 1990: 57) Friends who provide the kind of instrumental support usually only expected of kin were described as 'real' or 'true' friends or 'like a sister'.

Older people who are dying receive unbalanced care from friends. This friendship is bestowed as a gift and the very act of receiving the gift is gratifying to the giver. Jerrome writes:

> The cultural obsession with equity blinds us to the possibility of satisfactory inequitable relationships and the link between being able to receive and being a good friend.
>
> (1990: 62)

The existence of friends, whether as givers or receivers Jerrome argues, promotes self-esteem and self worth and so enhances a sense of well-being. Elaine Murphy has discussed the difficulties at the policy level of compensating for an intimate confiding relationship (1982). Whereas this may be beyond the scope of public policy the issue of providing instrumental support to dependent older people is one which crosses the public and private boundaries.

Malcolm Johnson in a discussion of dependency and interdependency points out that old age is frequently depicted as a time of dependency and that this is dichotomously set against the supposed independence of younger people. He believes that by virtue of being human we are all interdependent and such dichotomies are unhelpful:

> In complex societies the extent of interdependence is greatly increased. We are all totally dependent on many strangers (who produce food, power, clothing etc.) as well as on those with whom we live, work and have other personal relations. These forms of universal dependence are acknowledged, but not encompassed in the usage of the word. The logic for this appears to be that we are all contributors as well as receivers and thus equal partners in a social contract.
>
> (Johnson 1993: 258)

However there are those who are debarred from contributing in the economic sense. Many older people by virtue of compulsory retirement are in this category and therefore attract the label of dependency. As well as this 'structured dependency' older people are labelled dependent if they 'are incapable, temporarily or permanently, of performing a range of actions which are assumed to be within the competence of full citizens' (Johnson 1993: 259). If they are unable to carry out the normal activities of daily living such as washing, dressing, walking and talking then they are said to be heavily dependent. The ageist assumption that old age inevitably involves 'dependency' is challenged by Johnson and other gerontologists (Bytheway and Johnson 1990; Townsend 1981) as well as the notion that the 'inter' component of dependency necessarily stops if economic or physical dependency increases. Older people make up a large proportion of the 'givers' as well as the receivers of social support.

However, the increased risk of highly symptomatic chronic conditions in older people and especially women as they age, coupled with the increased likelihood of encountering bereavement, accompanied frequently with a loss of income, all indicate that instrumental and emotional support in old age is vital. At the same time the available pool of social support may, through death, marital break-up or geographical mobility be dwindling. Nevertheless the bulk of instrumental support given to older people is largely 'informal' and comes from kin.

There are important differences based on class, gender and ethnicity. Working class older women who had the lowest level of other resources identified by Taylor and Ford (1983) had the most resources in terms of social support. The greater geographical mobility of middle class people is thought to reduce the availability of immediate face to face support although other forms of contact such as telephone and letter writing are high.

In terms of gender, women throughout the life cycle establish smaller but more intimate social networks than men (Kessler et al. 1985) but men have larger networks which are most probably work related and therefore likely to diminish in old age. However because women live longer than men and because women have tended to marry men who are older than themselves they are more likely to be alone in old age whereas men are more likely to have a spouse to call on for instrumental support. This is complicated by the fact that women have more symptomatic conditions than men and so many men find themselves supporting a younger infirm wife. There is a widespread belief that older people from minority ethnic groups have the benefit of large extended families and supportive community networks. Whilst this may be the case for many, a range of studies of Asian and Afro-Caribbean families caution against too readily making this assumption (Barrow 1982; Ebrahim 1992; Blakemore and Boneham 1993; Gunaratnam 1993).

In times of adversity older people regardless of class, gender and ethnic differences will have to rely on informal networks for instrumental support. Much of this will come from kin and this informal care has received a great deal of attention in the last two decades. Having someone to take care of you when you are temporarily or permanently unable to care for yourself is of great personal concern. It makes the difference between being able to stay at home in familiar surroundings or having to go into an institution. And the spirit in which that care is given can make the difference between feeling loved and wanted as did Mr Jones or feeling rejected and a nuisance as Mr Healey did. At the end of one's life having someone to care for you because they care about you seems the ideal, but it is not always easily achieved. Mrs Healey by all accounts had cared about Mr Healey but she cared for him now with a mixture of resentment at his condition and bitterness that she did not have enough help either from other kin or from the statutory services. Caring for a chronically ill person can be a deeply rewarding experience, but it can also be a debilitating drain on one's own personal resources. Becoming a burden to others was identified in Chapters 2 and 4 as one of the things most older people fear and in studies that have looked at older people's attitudes to death and dying it is very rarely death itself that worries people, but the manner of their dying and more precisely the worry of becoming a burden (Sidell 1993).

The availability of informal care is not only a private resource, it is very much a public one (Henwood and Wicks 1984). Without it our health and welfare system would collapse. Qureshi and Walker write:

> the formal sector depends on informal carers: if only a small proportion of those with major caring responsibilities for frail elderly people – in excess of one million people (Henwood and Wicks 1984: 12) – metaphorically downed tools and ignored their emotions the personal social services would be swamped.
>
> (1989: 15)

Informal care was 'discovered' in the late 1970s in an effort to counter the widely held 'myth' that families in the western world, in contrast to earlier times and other cultural traditions, neglected their elderly kin. Feminists took up the issue setting it in the context of a critique of a sexual division of labour in which women's emotional labour in the domestic sphere went largely unrecognized and which disadvantaged them in the labour market and contributed to their economic dependence on men. In an effort to expose the very great burdens that carers experienced some of the early studies of caring presented a very negative view of informal care. These 'shock' tactics which I would argue were necessary at the time have recently attracted a good deal of criticism (Graham 1993; Morris 1993). Gunaratnam (1993) argues that they were the product of mainly white, middle class feminists and did not reflect the experience of minority ethnic groups in British society who might operate with other traditions. Another criticism is that they set the carers against the cared for (Campling 1981; Begum 1990), and, given that many of the older people being cared for were women, this was doing a good deal of harm to them. With hindsight this was an unfortunate by-product of what was intended as an attempt to make caring the concern of men as well as women and to put pressure on policy makers to provide 'care for the carers' (Finch and Groves 1983; Finch 1984; Henwood 1990a). A third criticism was that the early feminist writings on carers overstated the role of women and ignored the contribution of male carers. Arber and Gilbert (1989) have sought to redress this imbalance in the literature through their analysis of the 1980 General Household Survey (GHS) section on informal care. Unfortunately their analysis of the carers of severely disabled older people relates only to those living with their carer (co-residents) because the GHS did not explore the gender of the carers of severely disabled older people who live alone. From their analysis Arber and Gilbert write:

> Thus, the gender balance of co-resident caring for the elderly differs according to four types of kin relationship: (a) caring as part of a marital relationship – men and women are equally likely to care for an elderly spouse; (b) a filial relationship involving an unmarried carer – slightly fewer unmarried sons than unmarried daughters care for an elderly parent; (c) a sibling relationship – elderly sisters are much more likely to be carers than brothers; and (d) a filial relationship involving a married carer – we assume that men are unlikely to be carers ... Overall, therefore, although a majority of the carers of severely disabled elderly people are women, over one third of the co-resident carers are men.
>
> (Arber and Gilbert 1989: 114)

This is not so very different from the earlier work on carers which when those who did not live with the carer were taken into the equation, consistently found about 25 per cent of carers were male (Charlesworth *et al.* 1984; EOC 1980, 1982; Levin *et al.* 1988, 1983). Arber and Gilbert's analysis is important in emphasizing the caring work of older people mainly as spouses but also as siblings. A great deal of informal care is provided by old men and old women who may themselves be quite frail (Bytheway 1987).

Arber and Gilbert review the reasons why people care. For married couples the relationship will have gradually changed from one of reciprocity to one of dependency: 'The carer has "little choice" but to care and the transition to caring is often seen as "natural"' (Arber and Gilbert 1989: 115). Love was more likely to be the motive for caring when the carer had lived a long time with the older person but even if love was the original motive sometimes the burdens of caring tested that love beyond endurance, leading to situations like that of Mr and Mrs Healey. When an older person moves into the house of a child, and this is usually the daughter's home, Arber and Gilbert show that the motivation to care is more likely to be kinship obligation and a sense of duty which as they say is 'influenced by norms about gender obligations' (ibid.).

Whilst it is important to recognize that older male spouses and siblings provide care of the same quality and quantity of female spouses and siblings, the overall gender imbalance in caring has to be acknowledged. This is mainly due to the expectation on daughters to care. Qureshi and Walker in their survey of informal care point out that 'Among relatives it was primarily daughters who were bearing the physical and mental burdens of the whole range of caring and tending tasks' and 'It appears that with some exceptions, especially among husbands, men were able to choose which activities they helped with whereas female carers did not have such flexibility' (Qureshi and Walker 1989: 91, 92).

We tend to assume that older people themselves would always prefer to be cared for by kin if they should need help but evidence suggests that some older people would prefer to receive help from the statutory services rather than burden their children (Wenger 1984; Sixsmith 1986; Qureshi and Walker 1989), preferring to be cared about by their children than cared for.

Much of the thrust of feminist and other writers on informal care has been to mobilize resources to help carers and prevent a caring relationship from breakdown. This is motivated as much for the cared for as for the carer. Some have campaigned for monetary payments to be made to the person in need of care so that they can choose who should care for them and also be able to recompense their carer. Services under the umbrella of community care are supposed to provide a back up to informal care. The concept of community care and the policies which are derived from it are based on some fundamental assumptions about the nature and structure of family life. Gillian Dalley presents this argument:

> At the root of all community care policies seems to be the firm belief that the family is the appropriate unit and location for care. Privacy and independence – both regarded as goals to be prized and achieved – can best be secured by remaining in one's own home. The family, it is believed, has

a moral duty to care; the bosom of the family is the place where a dependent person 'ought' to be; the state should keep out of the essentially private business of caring wherever possible.

(Dalley 1988: 6)

She takes up the arguments put forward by Land and Rose (1985) that current community care policies create enforced dependency of the cared for on the family and compulsory altruism on the part of the carer. She criticizes these policies because they do not offer the carer the option of not caring and they do not offer choice to those in need of care. They also disadvantage those without family and for many older women this is increasingly the case. As she points out there is little of the dignity and independence much vaunted by proponents of community care for a confused older woman who is serviced by an array of different professionals, bussed to a local psychogeriatric day hospital each day and returned each evening to her own home where she sleeps and repeats the exercise the next day – 'the fact that the woman sleeps in a bed in her own home at night is deemed to represent own-home care' (Dalley 1988: 26).

At the heart of the debate about the relationship between formal and informal care and the partnership between family and state is a deeper ideological debate between what Barrett and McIntosh (1982) called familialism (and Gillian Dalley calls familism) and collectivism. Dalley argues that the ideology of familism 'has established its dominance and operates as a principle of social organization at both the domestic and public level, especially in the field of social care' (1988: 20). The social organization of daily living is based on the family as an ideological construct. This is not to imply that all or even most social organization adheres to that pattern but that it is the standard to be aspired to and against which all other forms of daily living are judged. Moreover it is the nuclear family as an 'ideal type' which is the model, if not the reality of most people's lives. The model prescribes very clear roles for men as providers and women as carers, thus setting up a sexual division of labour in both the private domestic world and the public world of work. The fact that household compositions are much more diverse than the nuclear type family structure and the fact that women in very large numbers work in the public world of work does not diminish the ideological strength of the model which sees the proper place for the care of dependent individuals as the home and women as innate carers.

The family is characterized as a 'haven in a heartless world' and a private form of protection against outside hostile forces and interference. Familist ideology is based on the wider philosophical tradition of possessive individualism with the related notions of self-determination, privacy and freedom of choice. In economic and political terms this is characterized by a free market economy based on the principles of *laissez-faire* with a minimum role for government.

The alternative ideology of collectivism puts great value on egalitarianism, but far from eschewing freedom, the collectivist view is that freedom must be available to all members of society. The freedom of one group should not be gained at the expense of the freedom of another. It is the role of the state to regulate those freedoms which if left to market forces will be counter to the value of egalitarianism. In matters of health and welfare a major distinction between individualism and collectivism hinges on matters of responsibility. Where does responsibility for health and the care of dependent people lie? Within a collectivist ideological framework such responsibility at the broadest level is societal, with the state responsible for the health and social care of all citizens. At the narrower level the local community, neighbourhood or group will have some responsibility for its members. Within an individualistic framework it is the individual and his/her immediate family who have the responsibility for his/her own health.

Fuelled by a fiscal crisis in the welfare state, but also because of growing disquiet at its former paternalistic and top down approach to care and fears that it fostered dependency and diminished human agency, a great deal of emphasis has been put on individual responsibility for health and the virtues of self care and personal health promoting lifestyles. Is this the way forward for the future and what are the prospects for a healthy 'old age'?

9
A healthy future for old age

Chronic illness and disability are not inevitable accompaniments of old age or even extreme old age and there is ample evidence, both quantitative and qualitative, to vouch for this. On the other hand it is the experience of too many older people whose mental, physical and social well-being are severely affected. Some older people remain trapped at the disease end of the health-ease-dis-ease continuum because they lack material, social or personal resources to move towards health. Others are helped by excellent medical treatment to feel 'healthy' in spite of their chronic illness. To achieve a healthy future for old age and promote the health of older people we need to pay attention both to preventing disease and to the treatment and management of chronic illness. In this chapter we will look at the policy implications for the public and private promotion of health in old age.

Inevitably as we approach the end of the century visions of the future are a favourite preoccupation. James Robertson (1993) suggests three directions for the future of industrialized societies. These are 'Business as usual', Hyper-Expansion (HE) and 'Sane, Humane and Ecological' (SHE). The 'Business as usual' postindustrial society will not be very different from the present but he sees HE and SHE futures as competing visions. The HE vision is one of expansion in science and technology. The SHE path represents a change of direction. The main values associated with these two visions he lists as follows:

HE	SHE
Quantitative values and goals	Qualitative values and goals
Economic growth	Human development
Organizational values and goals	Personal and interpersonal values and goals
Money values	Real needs and aspirations
Contractual relationships	Mutual exchange relationships

Business as Usual	HE	SHE
Individuals and society will continue to give lower priority to the promotion of health than to the treatment of sickness. Health services will continue to be primarily sickness services, and people's perception of themselves as consumers of those services will continue to dominate their perception of health. The main debate will continue to be whether sickness services should be provided commercially or at public expense.	Medical technology will solve most health problems. Genetic screening, organ transplants, new drugs, computer monitoring and computer records will eliminate or control congenital diseases and handicaps, enable the body to be maintained in good operating order, and enable expert physicians to deal more quickly and effectively than today with their patients' problems a widening range of which, such as bereavements, losses and failures, will become subject to medical treatment. Health promotion and sickness prevention may increase somewhat, but the increased dominance of medical experts and technologists will ensure that today's remedial bias remains strong.	Greater personal responsibility for health will lead people to the positive cultivation of their health and to the positive promotion of a healthy physical and social environment. Higher priority will be given to nutrition, public health and the psychosomatic aspects of health than is given today. Personal self-help and cooperative mutual aid in matters of health and sickness will be more highly rated than dependence on the expertise of health professionals. People will learn to manage the health hazards and stressful transitions in their lives. Nature and care will be emphasized, in contrast to the heroic interventionism of the HE future.

Figure 9.1 Robertson's vision for health
Source: Robertson 1993: 292

HE (*cont.*)
Intellectual, rational, detached
Masculine priorities
Specialization/helplessness
Technocracy/dependency
Centralizing

SHE (*cont.*)
Intuitive, experiential, empathetic
Feminine priorities
All-round competence
Self-reliance
Local

HE (cont.)	SHE (cont.)
Urban	Country-wide
European	Planetary
Anthropocentric	Ecological

Robertson is mainly concerned with the future of work, but he also presents his vision for health in Figure 9.1. Using Robertson's three possible futures as a framework we will examine some of the options for a healthy future for older people.

Business as usual

This option looks bleak for older people in the present climate of crisis in the welfare state. An expansion in health and welfare services in economic terms looks highly unlikely and a contraction of traditional services is firmly on the agenda. But the crisis in the welfare state is more than a fiscal crisis. Many people across the political spectrum are questioning the fundamental principles of welfare. The principle of universalism which is very dear to many older people who had first hand experience of selective benefits has come under attack. The goal of the Thatcher government was to free individuals from 'the shackles of compulsory welfare' which, it was argued, created welfare dependency and a levelling down rather than up in terms of equality. Seductive arguments about consumer choice and individual freedom have been pitted against equity and collectivism. Citizen's charters promised consumer sovereignty whilst at the same time a highly controlling government was eating away at locally provided services. Defenders of the welfare state and particularly the health services have not been uncritical of the top down paternalistic nature of many of our services and have argued for greater user participation. It seems very doubtful whether competitive tendering and market consumer led services will achieve this for many except the wealthiest members of society. However if health care is to continue to be provided at the public expense rather than commercially, the 'Business as usual' model is likely to involve cutting costs even further. Setting priorities or rationing is very much on the 'Business as usual' agenda and this will have profound effects on the health of older people.

The belief that the health services, after an initial period of high spending, would begin to cost less was clearly wrong and escalating costs have brought the issue of rationing into the public debate. Professor Alan Williams, an economist at York University, put the case for rationing health services in a radio programme saying:

> There are now so many beneficial things that the health care system can do for people that no country . . . can afford to do them all. So we have to . . . decide what are the things that we will do and what are the things that we can't really afford to do.
> ('Medicine Now', BBC Radio 4, 11 December 1986)

The issue of rationing raises very difficult ethical issues which we cannot fully do justice to here but I want to explore the attempt made by the University of York Centre for Health Economics (Gudex 1986) to find what they claim is an equitable way of rationing health resources and one which attempts to measure life's quality as well as its quantity. They devised the QALY or Quality Adjusted Life Year which is a form of cost-benefit analysis to be applied to any form of treatment. The costs of a treatment are likely to be much easier to measure than the benefits. Within a medical model of health adding to someone's years of life is a health benefit but the QALY measurement introduces the concern of quality into the added years.

For example if procedure A costs £420 and adds seven extra years of life one can work out how much each of these years costs. For procedure A it would be £60. If another procedure B, costs £600 and only adds six extra years of life, thus costing £100 per year, then it is clearly more costly than procedure A. But if procedure A leaves people immobile or in a good deal of pain and procedure B leaves people with no pain or mobility problems then it is clearly important to take that into account. The QALY is a well-year, not just an extra year, it is one free from disability or health related problems. One numerical year lived at less than free from disability or health related problems will be less than one QALY. The quality of the extra year is measured by a valuation matrix which takes into account an eight point disability rating with a four point distress rating.

The way the York economists reached a quality rating for the treatment procedures they measured has received a great deal of criticism (Fallowfield 1990) and many people are dismissive of the QALY. But we need to remember that decisions about the allocation of health resources have always been made, often by doctors or by faceless bureaucrats, in a fairly arbitrary way. The QALY represents an attempt to bring quality of life into the equation and to be concerned with fairness. However Weale (1988: 61) has pointed out that the QALY discriminates against certain groups of people, especially older people. He writes:

> any procedure that involves counting extra years of life as part of the benefit of medical procedures will risk shifting resources away from the elderly and towards younger age groups.

Also those whose quality of life before the procedure was low will be discriminated against even if there is subsequent improvement in their own quality of life. The effect of the QALY would be to divert resources away from those who most need them to those who could most benefit from them. This, Weale argues, is a fatal flaw in the QALY approach – it equates the concept of need with the ability to benefit. This runs counter to the demands of equity which require that those in greatest need should be allocated the greatest resources.

The QALY system of rationing is at least one which is open to scrutiny and can be argued against. Other more subtle forms of rationing like the decision not to screen older women routinely for breast and cervical cancer and decisions not to resuscitate certain older people need to be monitored. Also the moves to legalize voluntary euthanasia and to advocate 'living wills' raises some important anxieties about the implications such a move may have for older people, particularly older people with chronic illness and disability. In 1976 the European Federation for the Welfare of older people expressed such anxieties:

Table 9.1 Health care spending as a percentage of gross domestic product (GDP) 1985

	Public	Total
Australia	5.6	7.6
Austria	5.4	7.9
Belgium	5.6	7.3
Canada	6.5	8.6
Denmark	5.2	6.2
Finland	5.6	7.3
France	6.7	9.4
West Germany	6.3	8.1
Greece	4.1	4.2
Iceland	7.0	8.4
Ireland	7.0	8.0
Italy	6.2	7.4
Japan	4.8	6.6
Netherlands	6.6	8.3
Norway	6.3	6.6
Portugal	4.1	5.7
Spain	4.3	6.0
Sweden	8.4	9.3
Switzerland	5.4	7.9
United Kingdom	5.2	5.7
United States	4.4	10.8

Source: Schieber and Poullier (1987), cited in Weale (1988)

at some definable point in the future, national legislation may provide for or permit practices whose object is to put an end to the lives of old people allegedly incurable or incapable of improvement, who have become a burden on society.

(European CARITAS 1976)

Whilst the practice of voluntary euthanasia ostensibly increases the choices open to people over their own life and death, there is a fear that the 'temptation to move from voluntary assisted deaths to involuntary assisted death' would be very great (Twycross 1993: 157), and that there would be pressure on older people to seek voluntary euthanasia so as not to become a burden on relatives or society. Opponents of euthanasia also believe that the collective will to explore ways of relieving the symptoms of chronic illness and researching conditions which are at present incurable as well as emphasizing the importance of good palliative care for dying people will also be eroded by the widespread practice of euthanasia.

The fiscal crisis in welfare makes the 'Business as usual' future for health a worrying prospect for older people. The arguments that past levels of spending on the health services are not sustainable have been forceably put and seem to have widespread acceptance. Yet Britain spends a relatively small amount of GNP on health as the comparative Table 9.1 shows.

The NHS, without the vast bureaucracies of private insurance schemes, has been comparatively more efficient than the German or American systems of care. Comparing these various systems of health care on the basis of efficiency and equity and choice and control, Weale (1988) argues that the British system rates highly in terms of efficiency and equity and lower in terms of choice and control. Older people are acutely aware of the benefits the NHS has brought to their lives and the sense of security in knowing that they can call the doctor without worrying if they can afford to pay. This has also been identified as a major benefit of life in Britain by older black and minority ethnic older people and one which would persuade them to stay in spite of other problematic features of their lives. Those of us who take such benefits for granted need to beware of too easily dismissing the advantages of the NHS. Underresourcing and underfunding of the NHS should be vigorously opposed whilst at the same time attempting to change those aspects of the system which restrict and undermine the choice and control of the users of the system.

The HE future

What would the HE future offer older people? On the face of it, it promises an even longer and disease free life with new drugs to cure conditions such as arthritis and replacements for worn out organs and joints. And for future generations there is the possibility that control over our genes will eliminate the susceptibility to disease. What are the costs? In direct economic terms they are likely to be very high initially, even if there would be saving in the longer term. But in past experience this has not been the case. It seems unlikely that present public budgets would stand such expenditure. If such an expansion were left to market forces then the benefits would be unequally distributed on the basis of ability to pay, polarizing even more the present inequalities in health. Untrammelled expansion of medical technology raises many important ethical issues, not just about resource allocations, which should be subjected to much wider public and political debate. One such issue of Robertson's HE future which gives cause for concern is the greater dependence on medical experts and consequently a lessening of user control. This coupled with even greater medicalization of everyday life, such as defining grief as an illness reinforces the dominance of a medical model of health.

A grey area where there are gains and losses to be weighed of increasing medicalization is the menopause. A medical view of the menopause is to view it as a deficiency disease. The deficiency is of oestrogen which diminishes after women cease to be fertile. Hormone Replacement Therapy (HRT) has been developed which replaces the lost oestrogen and therefore makes up the deficiency. The claims for HRT have been lavish: firmer skin, lustrous hair, increases in energy levels including sexual energy, relief from depression and anxiety, protection from heart disease, reduction in vaginal dryness, relief from some of the unpleasant symptoms associated with the menopause such as 'hot flushes' and dizzy spells, but most importantly protection from osteoporosis. It is the last claim which has convinced many people that whatever else HRT may or may not do the prevention of brittle bones leading to fractures in later life is, for women, an undoubted benefit. HRT has many critics both inside and outside of the medical profession. Some of the criticisms are based on safety. In the early days of the use of HRT, large dosages of oestrogen alone used to be given and this was thought to increase the risk of uterine cancer. Lowering the dosage of oestrogen and adding the hormone progesterone is thought to have eliminated this risk. Evidence as to the increased risk of breast cancer is unclear with some research finding that HRT reduces the risk and others claiming that the risk is increased. Its confirmed ability to prevent osteoporosis, however, has convinced many doctors that it is of benefit to women past the child bearing years. Whilst it is of more benefit if started soon after the menopause it is still thought to be beneficial to older women in minimizing the risk of osteoporosis.

Many women's health groups are less convinced about the benefits of HRT and remain sceptical about its safety. They are wary of taking hormones over long periods of time after the experiences of the contraceptive pill and are not reassured by doctors. Opponents of HRT believe that natural remedies can also help prevent osteoporosis such as exercise and attention to diet. They believe that women need a lot more information about the pros and cons of HRT and the various alternatives in order that they should be able to make informed choices. This is the approach to health care which is implicit in the SHE future.

The SHE future

Robertson's SHE future is in complete contrast to the HE future, putting more emphasis on self-help and personal responsibility. It stresses the psychosomatic aspect of health, painting a much more holistic picture with less power invested in medical experts. Economically it seems a much more viable option, but where does it leave older people who still have to manage their health hazards and stressful life transitions? What help will they have and what about the health hazards which are outside of their control in the wider environment?

Many of the features of the SHE future are reflected in the concept of health promotion: greater personal responsibility for health, the cultivation of positive health, less dependence on experts and health professionals. The concept of health promotion was launched in the early 1980s by WHO and, as Malcolm Johnson pointed out, it has become the 'new gospel' (Johnson 1988). The stated aims of WHO were to promote 'health for all by the year 2000' (WHO, 1981, 1985). They identified the need for change both in the ways *and* conditions of people's lives. The emphasis was on both personal responsibility and public involvement in creating healthy lives and living conditions. People would be encouraged to take responsibility and participate in the development of their own health but governments were also encouraged to create environments conducive to health. The main tenets of the WHO's vision for health promotion were that:

- the basic resources for the health of any individual are income, shelter and food;
- people should fully participate in the development of their health;
- integrated action is required at different levels on factors influencing health – economic, environmental, social and personal;
- the focus should be on the reduction of inequalities in health;
- environments conducive to health should be developed;

- social networks and social ties should be strengthened;
- positive health behaviour and appropriate coping strategies should be encouraged;
- knowledge and information relating to health should be disseminated.

Translating this rhetoric into action is unlikely to be straightforward and the WHO was aware of some basic political and moral dilemmas in the strategy. They envisaged certain conflicts of interest at the social and individual level. These were:

1 Resources, including information, may not be accessible to people in ways which are sensitive or relevant to their expectations, beliefs, preferences or skills. This may increase social inequalities. Information alone is insufficient; raising awareness without increasing the degree of control or prospects for change may only succeed in generating anxieties and feelings of powerlessness.
2 Health promotion programmes are inappropriately directed at individuals at the expense of tackling economic and social problems. Policy makers often assume that people have the power completely to shape their own lives so as to be free from the avoidable burden of disease. Thus, when they are ill, they are blamed for this and discriminated against.
3 There is a danger that health promotion will be appropriated by one professional group and made a field of specialization to the exclusion of other professional and lay people. To increase control over their own health the public require a greater sharing of resources by professionals and government.
4 The risk of considering health as the ultimate goal, incorporating all life (a kind of 'healthism') with others prescribing what individuals should do for themselves and how they should behave.

(Kalache *et al.* 1988)

The reality of experience of health promotion activity in Britain over the last ten years has unfortunately fulfilled many of these fears. What are the consequences and prospects for older people?

The dissemination of health knowledge and information

One of the most important principles of the WHO concept of health promotion was its role in providing education and information on health issues. Knowledge and information are prerequisites for taking control over one's own health and for making informed choices about health. The dissemination of knowledge has been the cornerstone of the women's health movement and Chris Phillipson advocates a similar movement for health in old age:

> We need Age Well clinics, like the Well Woman clinics, which would prioritize older women; increase the status of the older person in the healing process; concentrate on sharing and interdependence; demystify medical knowledge.
>
> (1988: 16)

The women's health movement was a grass roots movement and it was women themselves who demanded more knowledge about their own bodies. We need to be wary of imposing knowledge and information on older people because they should know what is good for their health. Malcolm Johnson cautions:

> If our enthusiasms and innovations are to be truly helpful to older people, we have to listen to them and interpret what they say in the context of a whole life lived. We have to look more closely at the fit between what we believe will be good for others, and what they will accept and act upon.
> (1988: 14)

Some of the early preretirement education courses in the 1960s and 70s fell into the trap of lecturing to people about health in old age, with what amounted to a series of dos and don'ts. Allin Coleman who investigated the content and structure of such courses found three main areas of concern; these were:

1 The health component of the courses took the form of a formal lecture, usually given by a doctor with very little if any involvement of the participants.
2 The lecture was based on a medical model of health in old age and was highly prescriptive.
3 The doctor was given no briefing or support from the organizers of the course about the education needs or preferences of the participants.
(1992: 199)

In the early 1980s the then Health Education Council (HEC) funded a three year action research project carried out by the Centre for Health in Retirement Education (CHRE) to develop more effective models of health education for older people. This research aimed to change both the method of teaching and the content. Small group workshops were preferred to the lecture format so that participants could voice their own concerns as well as share their knowledge and experiences. They used a multidisciplinary approach in terms of educational input with nurses, health visitors, social workers, occupational therapists and physiotherapists as well as doctors as facilitators, and they sent out a questionnaire in advance of the workshops to find out the participants' needs. As well as giving information and the discussion of specific topics such as eyesight, blood pressure, joint and back problems and getting the best out of the NHS, they included skills training on how to cope with change. Because these courses were concerned with health and retirement it was important to focus on periods of transition and well-being in later life. A coping with change model was developed (Coleman and Chira 1991). The aim was to enable the participants to use their past experience of coping with change and relate this to the changes which retirement brought. Their intention was:

1 to analyse their understanding of change and transition;
2 to explore their feelings and reactions to change:
3 to consider the choices and options now before them:
4 to assess their skills in managing or coping with changes:
5 to identify the resources available to them to put their plans into action.
(Coleman 1992: 203)

Given that education was found by Colerick (1985), discussed in Chapter 7, to be important to the way older people coped with the changes and stresses they encountered in later life, this approach would seem to be helpful. Unfortunately such health courses for older people are not widely available (Meade 1988). Although all the courses on offer have been very well attended, they are unlikely to be able to reach large numbers of older people for various reasons such as mobility problems and lack of transport, lack of confidence in joining groups or simply lack of interest. Jane Tilston and Jude Williams (1992) see the over-75s health check in the GP's contract as an ideal opportunity for the giving and receiving of health information rather than simply carrying out a mechanical check. They cite a 'mini-survey' of pensioners who would welcome a health check that adopted a 'listening attitude', gave 'advice about treatment and health promotion' and took 'a broad approach to health and well-being'. Tilston and Williams conducted their own qualitative research with a group of older women into their priorities for health education programmes. The issues they identified included the following:

1 Ways of dealing with pain caused by arthritis and osteoarthritis which impinge on activity levels. Requests for sharing what is known about the management of pain . . .
2 Adequate information about what to expect from treatments, and about living with chronic conditions, so that people are prepared for the changes these bring, know what to expect, and what support is available . . .
3 Information that provides older women with scope for choice . . .
4 Information giving that acknowledges their fears – fear of what screening might reveal, particularly in terms of cancer screening; fear of doctors as authority figures . . .
5 Recognition that women who came to Britain as immigrants in the 1950s are now joining the ranks of senior citizens . . .
(Tilston and Williams 1992: 213, 214)

The last issue raises the question of health education which is sensitive both to age and ethnicity. Most hospitals and health centres in areas with a significant black and minority ethnic population provide literature in a range of languages but this does not indicate that the messages they convey are appropriate and sensitive to needs of that population. Most health education for older black and minority ethnic people is undertaken by local community groups. It is sporadic and tends to be one-off sessions. It is an area which has been neglected by health professionals (Pharoah and Redmond 1991). Esther Redmond, a health visitor specifically for older people in Lambeth, London liaised with a local Asian day centre for older people in the area and ran a series of groups for older Asian women to identify and meet their health education needs. She reports that 'the health visitor learned as well as advised, finding out about traditional remedies' (Pharoah and Redmond 1991: 22). She stressed the need to create a 'safe environment' in which to discuss sensitive issues such as health and identified factors which are likely to contribute to this. These included providing women only sessions, holding the sessions in their own community centre, having a trusted female member of their community present, making the programme relevant to their needs, and taking a sympathetic non-didactic approach (Pharoah and Redmond 1991: 22).

As well as age and ethnicity there is a gender issue to be addressed. Much health education seems either to target women specifically or tends to be taken up by women. The health education needs of older men might need special attention and the opportunity for men only sessions to encourage them to engage in such activities. This is important if the first of the pitfalls of health promotion is to be avoided.

Emphasis on individual behaviour rather than tackling economic and social problems

Changing individual lifestyles has been the message of much health promotion. Most of these messages have been directed to changing behaviours within a medical framework, 'stop smoking, drink less alcohol, eat less or different foods, cook with less fat, take regular exercise'. Without a wider attack on the social, economic and political conditions that largely determine an individual's choice of lifestyle, the end result is the 'victim blaming' which the WHO sought to avoid. Also as Malcolm Johnson argued the future health benefits from these changes in personal behaviours cannot be guaranteed in younger people so what do older people stand to gain from radically changing their lifestyle at 70 or 80? What incentive is there for a man of 75 with no obvious signs of lung disorder to give up smoking if he gets pleasure from this activity? Should a woman of 80 spread margarine on her bread when butter is a luxury she has only been able to afford in her old age? There is a dilemma. Clearly if changes in lifestyle are to be effective then the earlier they are started the better, but we should not fall into another trap of assuming that it is too late to change unhealthy lifestyles for older people. Exercise is now widely recognized to be beneficial to older people in reducing the fitness gap between the actual rate of decline in physical ability and the potential rate of decline (Muir Gray 1988). If exercise is to enhance health and well-being then it should be enjoyable and not forced onto people with stiff and painful joints. The opportunity for enjoyable and appropriate exercise is often a matter of access and the availability of facilities such as heated swimming pools. This is a matter of public policy and in order to avoid the dilemma envisaged by WHO, health promotion must be part of the public policy agenda at both the national and local level.

Healthy public policy

If we accept that 'the main causes of ill-health are socially, culturally and economically constructed and . . . are outside the individual's control' (Griffiths and Adams 1991: 221) then improvements in health will depend on changing environments which are harmful to health. As we discussed in Chapter 1 a more social model of health is concerned with creating environments which are conducive to health and which enable people to make health choices. This is very much the arena of public health as Draper claims, 'the core of public health action is avoiding or countering hazards in the environment' (1991: 7).

Public health in the past has had some spectacular successes in improving the health of the people. The nineteenth century separation of sewage from drinking water reduced dramatically the incidence of enteric diseases and the Clean Air Acts of the 1950s brought great improvements in levels of respiratory disease. Yet this environmental approach to health has been neglected and health has become the narrow preserve of medicine. Growing awareness of ecological issues has again focused attention on public health issues and the New Public Health Movement is concerned with both ecology and the social and economic conditions of people.

Given the established relationships between health, poverty, poor housing and education any attempt to promote the health of all individuals must address these issues. But there are other indirect areas of public policy which affect the health and well-being of individuals. Transport is one which is particularly important to older people. The lack of adequate public transport can render an older person housebound almost as effectively as arthritis. Crime is another issue which affects the health and well-being of older people. The fear of crime can hold many as prisoners in their own homes. The New Public Health Movement puts intersectorial working high on its agenda. In relation to governments this means that health issues cannot just be the concern of the Department of Health and neatly 'pigeon-holed' within one government department (Draper 1991: 17)

The Acheson Report of the Committee of Inquiry into the Future Development of the Public Health Function stressed that:

> the policies of almost every Government Department can have implications for health ... consequently there is a need for effective co-ordination of such policies if health is to be improved.
> (Acheson Report 1988: 2)

This coordination is necessary to avoid such situations as the health sector exhorting people to eat less fat while the agricultural sector is urging farmers to produce fatter cattle or creamier milk. Another example is the health sector's campaign against tobacco smoking whilst the rest of government refuses to ban cigarette advertising.

As well as putting health on the national public agenda the New Public Health Movement is concerned with policy at the local and regional level. A most important part of that policy is to enable people to participate in the policy initiatives that affect their lives. The National Community Health Resource aims to develop 'community health initiatives' which involve local informal groups of people coming together to tackle issues which effect their own health and well-being. There are examples of housing estates working to improve the quality of the environment and the lives of the residents such as the Pilton project in Edinburgh (Beattie, Jones and Sidell 1992). Amongst other activities the project runs stress management workshops, a keep-fit class for big women and a food co-op for the benefit of all its residents, young and old. Another type of interagency community health initiative was developed by Northampton District Health Authority specifically to combat social isolation in the rural areas of Northampton. Called the 'Right Angle Project', it operates two schemes specifically for older people: a day centre and luncheon club, and the

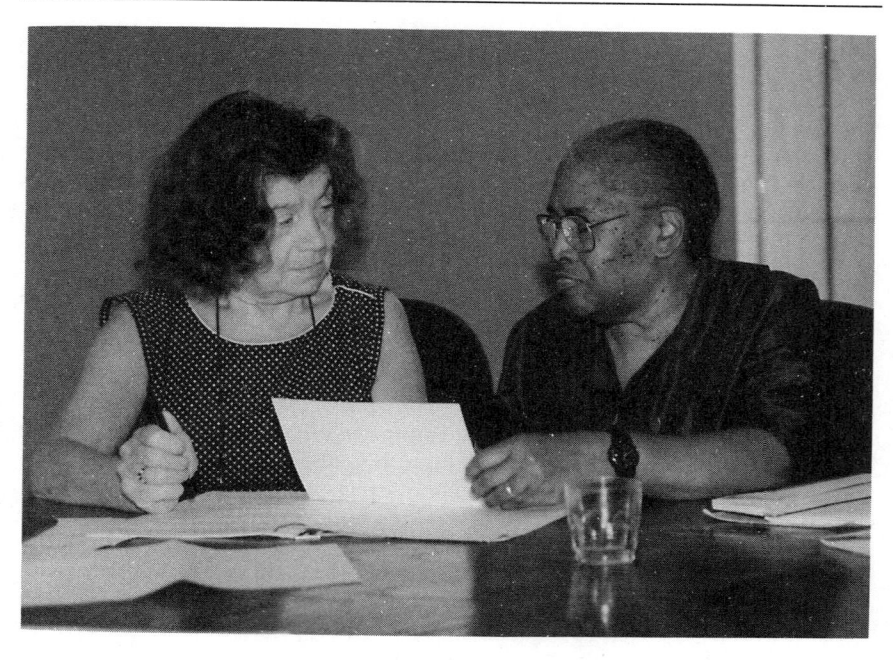

Workers on the Lewisham older women's project

Rural Wheels Scheme which is a volunteer transport system for mainly older people in isolated rural villages. Pensioners' groups have also identified transport as an issue on which to campaign and some groups are also active in direct health promotion like the Waterloo pensioners group who ran workshops on 'how to get the best out of your doctor' (Action for Health 1988). The Lewisham older women's project has identified health as an area for investigation. They are conducting a study of older women's views of the health services they receive in the borough, to give a voice to older women from a range of ethnic backgrounds, Vietnamese, Turkish, as well as Afro-Caribbean and Asian women whose voices are seldom heard.

Challenging the 'experts'

The fourth dilemma envisaged by the WHO that health promotion will be appropriated by one professional group to the exclusion of other professionals and lay people is particularly relevant in relation to older people. Challenging health professionals does not have a long tradition, particularly amongst older people. Yet Chris Phillipson believes that:

> the older patient's faith in 'the experts' is quite unjustified. 'Experts' are not necessarily expert; health professionals are not often trained in the problems of old age. They rely on stereotypes, and their advice is often designed to conceal ignorance. We need to challenge the concept of dependency on health-care professionals and emphasise the centrality of the patient.
>
> (1988: 16)

Good health education, community development projects and some of the self-health care initiatives discussed in Chapter 8 all aim to increase user participation and self-determination in health matters and represent a real challenge to health professionals. Specialized knowledge and skills are key elements in maintaining professional power and prestige. Ashton and Seymour (1993: 108) see potential areas of conflict between health professionals and the goals of WHO health promotion and the New Public Health movement:

> Professional power and prestige is contingent upon the acquisition of specific knowledge and skills which are exchanged for money in return for a service; the autonomy of the professional in the market is central as is his or her freedom to refuse a client. There is no commitment either to population coverage or to sharing power and demystifying knowledge. In this sense, there is a real conflict between the clinical model based on individual transactions and the public health model based on a social contract with entire communities. The consequence is that there is a great deal of rhetoric about public participation but a marked unwillingness to really engage in the processes which would bring it about.

The thrust of much of Robertson's SHE future for health is on personal autonomy and self-determination and this is in line with many of the criticisms of the NHS as paternalistic and undemocratic. Ironically this move towards participatory as opposed to paternalistic forms of welfare services has in Ashton and Seymour's view paved the way for the more 'victim blaming' view of individual responsibility for health and also 'made it possible for some governments to construe that the public no longer wants to have public services' (1993: 104).

Preserving the hard fought for benefits of universally available health services yet making them more accountable and sensitive to user's needs is clearly no simple matter. If a move towards the SHE future for health was motivated mainly by the fiscal crisis in the provision of welfare then we are in danger of losing what is best in the 'Business as usual' model. Similarly if the HE vision of an extension of medical technology was outside of the control of public accountability and availability then the potential for the abuse of power and control over the health and well-being of all individuals would be increased. Conversely medical technology put to the service of the health and well-being of older people for instance in eliminating a disease such as arthritis, would transform the lives of many older people and prevent much misery for future generations. The example of the technical advances in operations for cataracts gives reason not to reject the possible gains to be had from a properly controlled and available HE future.

The potential conflict between personal and public responsibility for health and the need to achieve a balance is mirrored by another potential conflict which is highlighted in Robertson's three visions of the future for health. That is the conflict between treatment and prevention and health promotion. However Ashton and Seymour (1993) argue that prevention and treatment should not be viewed in opposition to each other but rather as part of one whole health strategy. They also see treatment as preventative of ill-health and refer to it as tertiary prevention. Primary prevention and health promotion aim to prevent disorders before they occur, secondary prevention aims to detect disorders early in order to limit the course of the illness and prevent recurrence. Tertiary prevention they see as particularly relevant to older people, as it is

> aimed at reducing the burden of disability to the individual and to society and obtaining optimal health under the circumstances. Clearly, with an ageing population and in our current state of knowledge, there is a host of chronic conditions that we do not know how to prevent but where treatment may make all the difference to the quality of life and thus to health.
>
> (Ashton and Seymour 1993: 105)

Such tertiary prevention would include orthodox as well as non-orthodox treatment — anything that brought relief from pain and stiffness, that strengthened or compensated for social support, improved material circumstances or mobility either directly or through the provision of adequate and accessible public transport and any measures which might help prevent chronic illness resulting in a permanent state of dis-ease. Ashton and Seymour even go on to say that 'high quality terminal care is a form of tertiary prevention'. (1993: 105).

Primary and secondary prevention would if very successful produce a picture of health which would resemble Fries's compression of morbidity thesis (1980). Most people would reach the maximum biological lifespan and illness would be compressed into a very short period immediately before death. Baltes and Reichert believe that this is unlikely because it is, 'virtually impossible to create behavioural and environmental conditions that are optimal for all people' (1992: 251). Certainly we have not reached that state of affairs and chronic illness and disability is still likely to be the experience of many but certainly not all people at some stage in late life. Tertiary prevention offers the best hope of improving the health and well-being of many older people. Baltes and Reichart suggest a model of 'selective optimization with compensation' (p.237) to cope with an increase in biological vulnerability and an imbalance in the ratio of gains and losses' in later life. They suggest that by making selections between activities, perhaps increasing activities in some domains while decreasing other activities even to the point of becoming dependent and compensating or substituting skills for those which are lost, older people can optimize their physical, emotional and cognitive capacities. But they stress that in order for individuals to achieve this they require ageing-friendly environments which must be both prosthetic and stimulating at the same time. They should

> support and demand practice of functional systems even in old age. At the same time, however, environments are needed that are stress reducing or low-demanding.
>
> (Baltes and Reichert 1992: 252)

Unfortunately many older people experience extremely ageing-unfriendly or ageist environments and ironically it is often the pursuit of 'healthism' (the fourth of the WHO's potential dilemmas with health promotion) which contributes significantly to this ageist environment. There is a direct connection between 'healthism' and ageism. In the 'new gospel' of health and fitness the 'sinners' are the unfit. They are failures and the embodiment of what is to be avoided. Chronic illness and disability are shameful, to be hidden away and not admitted to, not because they cause pain and suffering, but because they render people incompetent by the standards of fitness aspired to by the rest of society. The temptation in trying to counter ageist attitudes is to minimize the prevalence of chronic illness and disability in old age and emphasize the fit and healthy old people. This only serves to reinforce the worship of fitness and adds to the disadvantage of those who do experience chronic illness and disability. We need to accept the challenge that chronic illness and disability bring, to try to prevent it by primary and secondary prevention, but to concentrate on tertiary prevention to relieve pain and suffering and help people live satisfying and valued lives maintaining a sense of well-being. More older people may then be enabled to move further towards the health end of the health-ease-disease continuum.

Bibliography

Aakster, C. (1986) Concepts in alternative medicine, *Social Science and Medicine*, 22(2), 265–73.
Acheson Report (1988) *Public Health in England.* The Report of the Committee of Enquiry into the future development of the Public Health Function. Cmnd. 289, London, HMSO.
Action for Health (1988) *Initiatives in Local Communities.* London, Community Projects Foundation.
Anderson, R. (1988) The quality of life of stroke patients and their carers. In R. Anderson and M. Bury (eds) *Living with Chronic Illness: The Experience of Patients and Their Families.* London, Unwin Hyman, pp. 14–42.
Anderson, R. and Bury, M. (eds) (1988) *Living with Chronic Illness: The Experience of Patients and Their Families.* London, Unwin Hyman.
Antonovsky, A. (1979) *Health, Stress and Coping: New perspectives on Mental and Physical Well-Being.* San Francisco, Jossey-Bass.
Antonovsky, A. (1984) The sense of coherence as a determinant of health. In J.P. Matarazzo (ed.) *Behavioral Health.* New York, Wiley.
Antonovsky, A. (1987). *Unravelling the Mystery of Health: How People Manage Others and Stay Well.* San Francisco, Jossey-Bass.
Arber, S. and Gilbert, N. (1989) Men: The forgotten carers, *Sociology*, 23(1), 111–18.
Arber, S. and Ginn, J. (1991a) Gender, class and income inequalities in later life. *British Journal of Sociology*, 42(3), 269–96.
Arber, S. and Ginn, J. (1991b) The invisibility of age: gender and class in later life. *The Sociological Review*, 39(2), 260–91.
Arber, S. and Ginn, J. (1991c) *Gender and Later Life – A Sociological Analysis of Resources and Constraints.* London, Sage Publications Ltd.
Arber, S. and Ginn, J. (1993) Gender and inequalities in later life, *Social Science and Medicine*, 26(1), 33–46.
Ashton, J. and Seymour, H. (1988) *The New Public Health.* Milton Keynes, Open University Press.
Ashton, J. and Seymour, H. (1993) The setting for a new public health. In A. Beattie, M.

Bibliography 165

Gott, L. Jones and M. Sidell (eds) *Health and Wellbeing: A Reader*. London, Macmillan. pp. 102–110.

Atkin, K. *et al.* (1989) Asian elders' knowledge of community, social and health services. *New Community*, 15(3), 439–45.

Backett, K. and Davison, C. (1992) Rationale or reasonable? Perceptions of health at different stages of life, *Health Education Journal*, 51/2.

Baltes, M.M. and Reichert, M. (1992) Successful ageing: The product of biological factors, environmental quality, and behavioural competence. In J. George and S. Ebrahim (eds) *Health Care for Older Women*, Oxford, Oxford University Press, pp. 236–53.

Barker, J. (1984a) Out in the cold, *Nursing Times*, 80(30), 19–20.

Barker, J. (1984b) *Black and Asian Old People in Britain*. London, Age Concern England.

Barker, A., Betmouni, S., Harrison, M. and Jones, R. (1992) Health checks for people over 75, *British Medical Journal* 305, 31 October.

Barrett, M. and McIntosh, M. (1982) *The Anti-social Family*. London, Verso.

Barrow, J. (1982) West Indian families: An insider's perspective. In R. Rapoport *et al.* (eds) *Families in Britain*. Routledge and Kegan Paul, pp. 220–32.

Beattie, A. (1993) The changing boundaries of health. In A. Beattie, M. Gott, L. Jones and M. Sidell (eds) *Health and Wellbeing: A Reader*. London, Macmillan.

Beattie, A. and Jones, L. (1993) Workbook 1, K256 *Health and Wellbeing*. Buckingham, Open University.

Beattie, A., Jones, L. and Sidell, M. (1992) *Health and Wellbeing*. K258, 2nd level distance learning course. Milton Keynes, Open University.

Bebbington, A.C. (1988) The expectation of life without disability in England and Wales, *Social Science and Medicine*, 27(4), 321–7.

Begum, N. (1990) *Burden of Gratitude: Women with Disabilities Receiving Personal Care*, University of Warwick, Social Care Practice Centre/ Department of Applied Social Studies.

Bennett, G.J. and Ebrahim, S. (1992) *The Essentials of Health Care of the Elderly*. London, Edward Arnold.

Berkman, L. and Syme, S. (1979) Social networks, host resistance and mortality. A nine-year follow up of Alameda County residents, *American Journal of Epidemiology*, 109, 186–204.

Bernard, M. (1985) *Health Education and Activities for Older People: A Review of Current Practice*, Working Papers on the Health of Older People No. 2. Health Education Council, in association with the Department of Adult Education, Keele, University of Keele.

Bernard, M. (1988) Taking charge: Strategies for self-empowered health behaviour amongst older people, *Health Education Journal*, 47(2/3), 87–90.

Bernard, M. (1989) Research in action: Self-health care and older people, *Hygie-International Journal of Health Education*, 8(2), 11–15.

Bernard, M. and Ivers, V. (1986) Peer health counselling: A way of countering dependency? In C. Phillipson *et al.* (eds) *Dependency and Interdependency in Old Age: Theoretical Perspectives and Policy Alternatives*. London, Croom Helm, pp. 288–99.

Bhalla, A. and Blakemore, K. (1981) *Elders of the Ethnic Minority Groups*. Birmingham, AFFOR (All Faiths for One Race).

Blakemore, K. (1982) Health and illness among the elderly of minority ethnic groups living in Birmingham: Some new findings, *Health Trends*, 14, 69–72.

Blakemore, K. (1983) Ethnicity, self-reported illness and use of medical services by the elderly, *Postgraduate Medical Journal*, 59, 668–70.

Blakemore, K. and Boneham, M. (1993) *Ageing and Ethnicity*, Buckingham, Open University Press.

Blaxter, M. (1983) The causes of disease, women talking, *Social Science and Medicine*, 17(2), 59–69.

Blaxter, M. (1990) *Health and Lifestyles*, London, Routledge.

166 Bibliography

Blaxter, M. (1993) 'Why do the victims blame themselves?' In A. Radley (ed) *Worlds of Illness*. London, Routledge. pp. 124–42.

Blaxter, M. and Paterson, L. (1982) *Mothers and Daughters: A Three-generational Study of Health, Attitudes and Behaviour*. Oxford, Heinemann Educational.

Blazer, D. (1982) Social support and mortality in an elderly community population, *American Journal of Epidemiology*, 115, 684–94.

Bosanquet, N. and Gray, A. (1989) 'Will you still love me? New opportunities for health services for elderly people in the 1990s and beyond', National Association of Health Authorities (NAHA) Research Paper No. 2, Birmingham, NAHA.

Bowling, A. (1991) *Measuring Health: A Review of Quality of Life Measurement Scales*. Milton Keynes, Open University Press.

Brown, G. and Harris, T. (1978) *The Social Origins of Depression*. London, Tavistock.

Burns, B. and Phillipson, C. (1986) *Drugs, Ageing and Society: Social and Pharmacological Perspectives*. London, Croom Helm.

Burns, B. and Phillipson, C. (1988) Elderly People and drug based therapy, In B. Gearing, M. Johnson and T. Heller (eds) *Mental Health Problems in Old Age*. Chichester, Wiley, pp. 198–209.

Bury, M. (1982) Chronic illness as biographical disruption, *Sociology of Health and Illness*, 4, 167–82.

Bury, M. (1988a) Arguments about ageing: long life and its consequences. In N. Wells and C. Freer (eds) *The Ageing Population: Burden or Challenge?* London, Macmillan, p. 173.

Bury, M. (1988b) Meanings at risk: The experience of arthritis, In R. Anderson and M. Bury (eds) *Living with Chronic Illness: The Experience of Patients and Their Families*. London, Unwin Hyman, pp. 89–116.

Bury, M. (1991) The sociology of chronic illness: A review of research and prospects, *Sociology of Health and Illness*, 13(4), 451–67.

Bury, M. and Holme, A. (1991) *Life After Ninety*, London, Routledge.

Butler, R.M. (1963) The life review: An interpretation of reminiscence in the aged, *Psychiatry*, 26, 65–76.

Bytheway, B. (1982) Fries and Crapo review symposium – Ageing and the rectangular survival curve, *Ageing and Society*, 2(2), 389–91.

Bytheway, B. (1987) Male carers: Questions of intervention, in J. Twigg (ed.) *Evaluating Support to Informal Carers*. York: University of York Social Policy Research Unit.

Bytheway, B., Keil, T., Allatt, P. and Bryman, A. (eds) (1989) *Becoming and Being Old: Sociological Approaches to Later Life*. London, Sage.

Bytheway, B. and Johnson, J. (1990) On defining ageism, *Critical Social Policy*, 29, 27–39.

Calnan, M. (1987) *Health and Illness*, London, Tavistock.

Campling, J. (ed.) (1981) *Women with Disabilities: Images of Ourselves*, London, Routledge.

Caplan, G. (1974) *Social Support and Community Mental Health*. New York, Basic Books.

Cassel, J. (1976) The contribution of the social environment to host resistance, *American Journal of Epidemiology*, 104, 107–23.

Chadwick, D., Gillart, D.A., Gingell, J.C. and Abrams, P.H. (1990) Screening for carcinoma of the prostate, *British Medical Journal*, 301, 14 July, 119–20.

Chadwick, E. (1842) *Report on the Sanitary Condition of the Labouring Population of England*, Vol. 26. London, HMSO.

Charlesworth, A. Wilkin, D. and Durie, A. (1984) *Carers and Services: A Comparison of Men and Women Caring for dependent Elderly People*. Manchester, Equal Opportunities Commission.

Charmaz, K. (1983) Loss of self: A fundamental form of suffering in the chronically ill, *Sociology of Health and Illness*, 5, 168–95.

Charmaz, K. (1990) Discovering chronic illness: Using grounded theory, *Social Science and Medicine*, 30(11), 1161–72.

Cipolla, C. (1973) *Cristofano and the Plague: A Study of Public Health in the Age of Galileo.* London, Collins.
Cockerham, W.C. et al. (1983) Ageing and perceived health status, *Journal of Gerontology*, 38, 349–55.
Cohen, S. and Wills, T.A. (1985) Stress, social support, and the buffering hypothesis, *Psychological Bulletin*, 98(2), 310–57.
Coleman, A. (1992) Pre-retirement education and the role of the GP. In J. George and S. Ebrahim (eds) *Health Care for Older Women.* Oxford, Oxford University Press, pp. 197–204.
Coleman, A. and Chira, T. (1991) *Coping with Change – Focus on Retirement.* London, Health Education Authority.
Coleman, P. (1993) Adjustment in later life. In J. Bond, P. Coleman and S. Peace (eds) *Ageing in Society.* London: Sage.
Colerick E.J. (1985) Stamina in later life, *Social Science and Medicine*, 21(9), 997–1006.
Coni, N., Davison, W. and Webster, S. (1992) *Ageing: The Facts.* 2nd edn, Oxford, Oxford University Press.
Coppard, L.C. et al. (1984) *Self-health Care and Older People – A Manual for Public Policy and Programme Development.* Copenhagen, World Health Organization.
Cornwell, J. (1984) *Hard Earned Lives: Accounts of Health and Illness from East London.* London, Tavistock.
Cornwell, J. (1989) *The Consumers' View: Elderly People and Community Health Services.* London, King's Fund Centre.
Cornwell, J. and Gearing, B. (1989) Doing biographical reviews with older people, *Oral History*, 17(1), Spring.
Coward, R. (1989) *The Whole Truth: The Myth of Alternative Health.* London, Faber and Faber.
Cox, B.D. et al. (1987) *The Health and Lifestyles Survey.* London, The Health Promotion Research Trust.
Cruickshank, J.K., Beevers, D.G., Osbourne, V.L., Haynes, R.A., Corlett, J.C.R. and Selby, S. (1980) Heart attacks, stroke, diabetes and hypertension in West Indians, Asians and whites in Birmingham, England, *British Medical Journal*, 281, 25 October, 1108.
Cumming, E. and Henry, W.E. (1961) *Growing Old: The Process of Disengagement.* New York, Basic Books.
Dalley, G. (1988) *Ideologies of Caring: Rethinking Community and Collectivism.* Houndmills, Macmillan Educational Ltd.
Dean, K. (1982) Self-care: What people do for themselves. In S. Hatch and I. Kickbusch (eds) *Self-Help and Health in Europe – New Approaches in Health Care.* Copenhagen, World Health Organization, pp. 20–31.
Dean, K. (1986) Social support and health: pathways of influence. *Health Promotion* 1, 133–50.
Dean, K. et al. (1986) *Self-Care and Health in Old Age.* London, Croom Helm.
Department of Health and Social Security (DHSS) (1987) *Hospital In-Patient Enquiry, 1985*, Series MB4, No. 27, London, HMSO.
Department of Health and Social Security (DHSS) (1989) *Mental Health Statistics for England 1986.* London, HMSO.
Dohrenwend, B.S. and Dohrenwend, B.P. (1974) *Stressful Life events: Their Nature and Effects.* New York, Wiley.
Donovan, J. (1986) *We Don't Buy Sickness It Just Comes.* Aldershot, Gower Publishing Group Ltd.
Doyal, L. (1979) *The Political Economy of Health Care.* London, Pluto Press.
Draper, P.(ed.) (1991) *Health Through Public Policy: The Greening of Public Health.* London, Green Print.

Dubos, R. (1961) *Mirage of Health*. New York, Andor Books.
Dubos, R. (1971) *Man Adapting*. New Haven, Yale University Press.
Ebrahim, S. (1992) Health of elderly Asian women. In J. George and S. Ebrahim (eds) *Health Care for Older Women*. Oxford, Oxford University Press, pp. 168–78.
Ebrahim, S. and Hillier, S. (1991) Ethnic minority needs, *Reviews in Clinical Gerontology*, 1, 195–9.
Ebrahim, S., Smith, C. and Giggs, J. (1987) Elderly immigrants – a disadvantaged group? *Age and Ageing*, 16(4), 249–55.
Ebrahim, S., Patel, N., Coats, M., Greig, C., Gilley, J., Bangham, C. and Stacey, S. (1991) Prevelance and severity of morbidity among Gujarati Asian-elders: a controlled comparison. *Family Practice*, 8(1), 57–62.
Equal Opportunities Commission (EOC) (1980) *The Experience of Caring for Elderly and Handicapped Dependants: Survey Report*. Manchester, EOC.
Equal Opportunities Commission (EOC) (1982) *Who Cares for the Carers?*. Manchester, EOC.
Erikson, E. (1965) *Childhood and Society*. Harmondsworth, Penguin (first published 1950).
Estes, C.L., Gerard, L.E., Zones, J.S. and Swan, J.H. (1984) *Political Economy, Health and Ageing*. Boston, Little Brown.
European CARITAS (1976) Working Party on old people. Memorandum, European Federation for the Welfare of the Elderly. *Newsletter*, March 1976, 511.
Evers, H. (1983) Elderly women and disadvantage. In D. Jerrome (ed.) *Ageing in Modern Society*. London, Croom Helm, pp. 25–44.
Evers, H. (1985) The frail elderly woman: Emergent questions in ageing and women's health. In E. Lewin and V. Oleson (eds) *Women, Health and Healing: Towards a New Perspective*. London, Tavistock, pp. 86–112.
Evers, H. (1993) The historical development of geriatric medicine as a speciality. In J. Johnson and R. Slater (eds) *Ageing in Later Life*. London, Sage.
Fallowfield, L. (1990) *The Quality of Life: The Missing Measurement in Health Care*. London, Souvenir Press.
Fennell, G., Phillipson, C. and Evers, H. (1988) *The Sociology of Old Age*. Milton Keynes, Open University Press.
Fennell, G., Emerson, A.R., Sidell, M. and Hague, A. (1981) *Day Centres for the Elderly in East Anglia*. Norwich, Centre for East Anglia Studies.
Ferraro, K.F. (1987) Double jeopardy to health for black older adults? *Journal of Gerontology*, 42(5), 538–53.
Finch, J. (1984) Community care: Developing non-sexist alternatives, *Critical Social Policy*, 9, 6–18.
Finch, J. and Groves, D. (eds) (1983) *A Labour of Love: Women, Work and Caring*. London, Routledge and Kegan Paul.
Finkelstein, V. (1993) Disability: A social challenge or an administrative responsibility? In J. Swain, V. Finkelstein, S. French and M. Oliver (eds) *Disabling Barriers – Enabling Environments*, London, Sage.
Fletcher, A. (1992) Controversies in screening for breast and cervical cancer. In J. George and S. Ebrahim (eds) *Health Care for Older Women*, Oxford, Oxford University Press, pp. 222–35.
Ford, G. and Taylor, R. (1985) The elderly as underconsulters: A critical reappraisal. *Journal of the Royal College of General Practitioners*, 35, 244–64.
Fox, A.J. and Goldblatt, P.O. (1982) *Longitudinal Study: Socio-Demographic Mortality Differentials*. Series LS No. 1, OPCS, London, HMSO.
Fox, A.J., Jones, D., Moser, I.R. and Goldblatt, P. (1985) Socio-economic differences in mortality, *Population Trends*, 40, 10–16.
Freer, C.B. (1985) Geriatric screening: A reappraisal of the preventive strategies in the care of the elderly. *Journal of the Royal College of General Practitioners*, 35, 288–90.

Fries, J.F. (1980) Ageing, natural death and the compression of morbidity, *New England Journal of Medicine*, 303(3), 130–35.
Fulder, S. (1988) *The Handbook of Complementary Medicine*, 2nd edn. Oxford: Oxford University Press.
Gearing, B. and Dant, T. (1990) Doing biographical research. In S.M. Peace (ed) *Researching Social Gerontology: Concerns, Methods and Issues*. London, Sage, pp. 143–59.
Gee, E.M. and Kimball, M.M. (1987) *Women and Ageing*. Toronto, Butterworths.
George, C. (1981) The effect of age on drug metabolism. *MIMS Magazine*, 1 March, 55–9.
George, J. and Ebrahim, S. (eds) (1992) *Health Care for Older Women*. Oxford, Oxford University Press.
Glendenning, F. and Pearson, M. (1988) *Black and Ethnic Minority Elders in Britain: Health Needs and Access to Services*, Working Papers on the Health of Older People, No. 6. Health Education Authority in association with the Centre for Social Gerontology, Keele, University of Keele.
Goffman, E. (1963) *Stigma: Notes on the Management of Spoiled Identity*. Harmondsworth, Penguin.
Gove, E.R. (1973) Sex, marital status and mortality. *American Journal of Sociology*, 79, 45–67.
Gove, W. (1984) Gender differences in mental and physical illness: The effects of fixed roles and nurturant roles, *Social Science and Medicine*, 1, 77–91.
Gove, W. and Hughes, M. (1979) Possible cause of the apparent sex differences in physical health: An empirical investigation. *American Sociological Reviews*, 44, 126–46.
Graham, H. (1993) Feminist perspective in caring. In J. Bornat, C. Pereira, D. Pilgrim, and F. Williams (eds) *Community Care: A Reader*. London, Macmillan, pp. 124–33.
Griffiths, J. and Adams, L. (1991) The new health promotion. In P. Draper (ed.) *Health Through Public Policy: The Greening of Public Health*. London, Green Print.
Gudex, C. (1986) 'QALYS' and their use by the health service: Discussion paper? University of York Centre for Health Economics: 14.
Gunaratnam, Y. (1993) Breaking the silence: Asian carers in Britain. In J. Bornat, C. Pereira, D. Pilgrim, and F. Williams (eds) *Community Care: A Reader*. London, Macmillan, pp. 114–23.
Hannay, D.R. (1978) Symptom prevalence in the community, *Journal of the Royal College of General Practitioners* 28, 492–9.
Hannay, D.R. (1979) *The Symptom Iceberg: A Study of Community Health*. London, Routledge and Kegan Paul.
Hardman, A. (1992) Exercise and older women. In J. George and S. Ebrahim (eds) *Health Care for Older Women*, Oxford, Oxford University Press, pp.222–35.
Hart, N. (1985) *The Sociology of Health and Medicine*. Ormskirk, Causeway Books.
Havighurst, R.J. (1963) Successful aging. In R.H. Williams *et al.* (eds) *Processes of Aging*, Vol. 1, New York, NY, Atherton, pp. 299–320.
Henwood, M. (1990a) *Community Care and Elderly People – Policy, Practice and Research Review*. London, Family Policy Studies Centre.
Henwood, M. (1990b) No sense of urgency. In E. McEwan (ed.) *Age: The Unrecognised Discrimination*. London, Age Concern England, pp. 43–57.
Henwood, M. (1993) Age discrimination in health care, In J. Johnson and R. Slater (eds) *Ageing and Later Life*. London, Sage, pp. 112–19.
Henwood, M. and Wicks, M. (1984) *Forgotten Army*. Family Care and Elderly People Briefing Paper, London, Family Policy Studies Centre.
Herzlich, C. (1973). *Health and Illness: A Social Psychological Analysis*. London, Academic Press.
Hickey, T. (1986) Health behaviour and self-care in late life: An introduction. In K. Dean, T. Hickey and B.E. Holstein (eds) *Self-care and Health in Old Age*. London, Croom Helm.

Holmes, T.H. and Rahe, R.H. (1967) The social maladjustment rating scale, *Journal of Psychosomatic Research*, 11, 213–18.
Hoyes, L. and Means, R. (1993) Markers, contracts and social care services: prospects and problems, In J. Bornat, C. Pereira, D. Pilgrim and F. Williams (eds) *Community Care: A Reader*. London, Macmillan, pp. 276–86.
Isaacs, B., Livingstone, M. and Neville, Y. (1972) *Survival of the Unfittest: A Study of Geriatric Patients in Glasgow*. London, Routledge and Kegan Paul.
Ivers, V. and Meade, K. (1991) *Older Volunteers and Peer Health Counselling: A New Approach to Training and Development*. Stoke-on-Trent, The Beth Johnson Foundation.
Jamieson, A. (1989) A new age for older people? Policy shifts in health and social care, *Social Science and Medicine*, 29(3), 445–54.
Jerrome, D.M. (1981) The significance of friendship for women in later life, *Ageing and Society*, 1(2), 175–84.
Jerrome, D.M. (1990) Frailty and friendship, *Journal of Cross-cultural Gerontology*, 5(1), 51–64.
Jerrome, D.M. (1991) Loneliness: Possibilities for intervention, *Journal of Aging Studies*, 5(2), 195–208.
Johnson, M. (1993) Dependency and Interdependency, In J. Bond, P. Coleman and S. Peace (eds) *Ageing and Society*, 2nd edn. London, Sage.
Johnson, M.L. (1988) Health promotion and older people: Policy and provision. In J. Groombridge (ed.) *Health Promotion and Older People*. London, CHRE, pp. 8–15.
Jones, D. (1992) Informal care and community care. In J. George and S. Ebrahim (eds) *Health Care for Older Women*, Oxford, Oxford University Press, pp. 16–26.
Kalache, A., Warnes, A.M. and Hunter, D.J. (1988) *Promoting Health among Elderly People*, London, King Edward's Hospital Fund for London.
Kasl, S. (1983) Social and psychological factors affecting the course of a disease: an epidemiological perspective, in D. Mechanic (ed.) *Handbook of Health, Health Care and the Health Professions*. New York, Free Press, pp. 683–708.
Kessler, R., McLeod, J. and Wethington, E. (1985) The costs of caring: A perspective on the relationship between sex and psychological distress. In I. Sarason and B. Sarason (eds) *Social Support: Theory, Research and Applications*. Dordrecht, The Netherlands, Nijhoff.
Kitwood, T. (1993) Towards a theory of dementia care: the interpersonal process. *Ageing and Society*, 13(1): 51–67.
Kobasa, S.C., Maddi, S.R. and Corrington, S. (1981) Personality and constitution as mediators in the stress-illness relationship, *Journal of Health and Social Behaviour*, 22, 368–78.
Kobasa, S.C., Maddi, S.R. and Kahn, S. (1982) Hardiness and health: A prospective study. *Journal of Personality and Social Psychology*, 42(1), 168–77.
Lalonde, M. (1974) *A New Perspective on the Health of Canadians*. Ottawa, Ministry of Supply and Services.
Land, H. and Rose, H. (1985) Compulsory altruism for some or an altruistic society for all? In P. Bean, J. Ferris and D. Whynes (eds) *In Defence of Welfare*. London, Tavistock.
Lazarus, R.S. (1966) *Psychological Distress and the Coping Process*. New York, NY, McGraw-Hill.
Lazarus, R.S. and Launier, R. (1978) Stress-related transactions between person and environment. In L.A. Pervin and M. Lewis (eds) *Perspectives in interactional psychology*. New York, Plenum.
Levin, E., Sinclair, I. and Gorbach, P. (1988) *Families, Services and Confusion in Old Age*. Aldershot, Gower.
Lewis, M. (1985) Older women and health: An overview. In S. Golub and R.J. Freedman (eds) *Health Needs of Women As They Age*. New York, NY, Haworth Press, pp. 1–16.
Lewith, G. and Aldridge, D. (1991) *Complementary medicine and the European Community*. Saffron Walden, The C.W. Daniel Company.

Bibliography 171

Lowenthal, M.F. (1965) Antecedents of isolation and mental illness in old age, *Archives of General Psychiatry*, 12, 245–54.

MacIntyre, S. (1977) Old age as a social problem. In R. Dingwall, C. Heath, M. Reid and M. Stacey (eds) *Health Care and Health Knowledge*. London, Croom Helm, pp. 41–63.

McKeown, T. (1976) *The Role of Medicine – Dream, Mirage or Nemesis*, London, Nuffield Provincial Hospital Trust.

Mahoney, F.I. and Barthel, D.W. (1965) Functional evaluation: The Barthel Index, *Maryland State Medical Journal*, 14, 61–65.

Marcus, A.C. and Seeman, T.E. (1981) Sex differences in reports of illness and disability: A preliminary test of the 'fixed role obligations' hypothesis, *Journal of Health and Social Behaviour*, 22, 174–82.

Marmot, M.G., Adelstein, A. and Bulusu, L. (1983) Immigrant mortality in England and Wales, *Population Trends*, 33, 14–17.

Marmot, M.G., Adelstein, A. and Bulusu, L. (1984) Immigrant mortality in England and Wales, 1970–78: causes of death by country of birth, *Studies on Medical and Population Subjects*, No. 47, London, HMSO.

Martin, J., Meltzer, H. and Elliot, D. (1988) *The Prevalence of Disability Among Adults. OPCS Surveys of Disability in Great Britain, Report No. 1*. London, HMSO.

Maslow, A. (1954) *Motivation and Personality*, New York, Harper and Row.

Meade, K. (1988) Health Courses for Pensioners. In J. Groombridge (ed.) *Health Promotion and Older People*. London, CHRE, pp. 28–31.

Mieson, B. (1992) Attachment theory and dementia. In G.M.M. Jones and B. Mieson (eds) *Care-giving in Dementia: Research and Applications*. London, Routledge.

Moen, E. (1978) The reluctance of the elderly to accept help, *Social Problems*, 25, 3.

Morris, J. (1993) 'Us' and 'Them'? Feminist research and community care. In J. Bornat, C. Pereira, D. Pilgrim, and F. Williams (eds) *Community Care: A Reader*. London, Macmillan, pp. 156–66.

Muir Gray, J.A. (1988) Health and the individual. In J. Groombridge (ed.) *Health Promotion and Older People*. London, CHRE, pp. 21–24.

Murphy, E. (1982) Social origins of depression in old age, *British Journal of Psychiatry*, 141, 135–42.

Murphy, E. (1988) Prevention of depression and suicide. In B. Gearing et al. (eds) *Mental Health Problems in Old Age*, Chichester, John Wiley and Sons Ltd, pp. 67–73.

Nathanson, C.A. (1975) Illness and the feminine role: A theoretical review, *Social Science and Medicine*, 9, 57–62.

Nathanson, C.A. (1977) Sex, illness and medical care: A review of data, theory and method, *Social Science and Medicine*, 11(1), 13–25.

Norman, A. (1985) *Triple Jeopardy: Growing Old in a Second Homeland*. London, Centre for Policy on Ageing.

Office of Population Censuses and Surveys (OPCS) (1987) *Hospital Inpatient Enquiry: 1985* London, OPCS.

Office of Population in Censuses and Surveys (OPCS) (1988) *General Household Survey 1985*, London, OPCS.

Office of Population Censuses and Surveys (OPCS) (1989) *Mortality Statistics 1986, England and Wales*. DH1 No. 18, London, HMSO.

Office of Population Censuses and Surveys (OPCS) (1990) Population Trends, 62. London, HMSO.

Office of Population Censuses and Surveys (OPCS) (1993) *General Household Survey 1991*. London, OPCS.

Oliver, M. (1990) *The Politics of Disablement*. London, Macmillan.

Ooijendijk, W.T.M., Mackenbach, J.P. and Limberger, H.H.B. (1981) *What is Better? An investigation into the use of, and satisfaction with, complementary and official medicine in the Netherlands*. London, Threshold.

Parsons, T. (1951) *The Social System*. Glencoe, Illinois, Free Press.

Passant, H. (1990) A holistic approach in the ward, *Nursing Times* 86, 24 January, 26–28.

Paykel, E.S. (1974) Life stress and psychiatric disorder: Applications of the chemical approach. In B.S. Dohrenwend and B.P. Dohrenwend (eds) *Stressful Life Events: Their Nature and Effects*. New York, Wiley and Sons, pp. 135–49.

Pearlin, L.I. and Schooler, C. (1978) The structure of coping, *Journal of Health and Social Behaviour*, 19, 2.

Pearson, A. and Vaughan, A. (1986) *Nursing Models for Practice*. London, Heineman.

Pearson, M. (1991) Care of black and ethnic minority elders. In S.J. Redfern (ed) *Nursing Elderly People*. 2nd edn, Edinburgh, Churchill Livingstone, pp. 437–47.

Pharoah, C. and Redmond, E. (1991) Care for ethnic elders. *Health Service Journal*, 16 May: 20–22.

Phillips, D.L. and Segal, B.E. (1969) Sexual symptoms and psychiatric symptoms, *American Sociological Review*, 34, 58–72.

Phillipson, C. (1988) Health professionals and health promotion. In J. Groombridge (ed.) *Health Promotion and Older People*. London, CHRE, pp. 15–17.

Pilgrim, D. and Rogers, A. (1993) *A Sociology of Mental Illness*. Buckingham: Open University Press.

Pill, R. and Stott, N.C.H. (1981) Relationship between health locus of control and belief in the relevance of lifestyle to health, *Patient Counselling and Health Education*, 3, 95–9.

Pill, R. and Stott, N.C.H. (1982) Concept of illness causation and responsibility: Some preliminary data from a sample of working-class mothers, *Social Science and Medicine*, 16, 43–52.

Pill, R. and Stott, N.C.H. (1985) Preventive procedures and practices among working-class women: New data and fresh insights, *Social Science and Medicine*, 21, 975–83.

Pinder, R. (1988). 'Striking balances: Living with Parkinson's disease, In R. Anderson and M. Bury (eds) *Living with Chronic Illness: The Experience of Patients and Their Families*. London, Unwin Hyman, pp. 67–88.

Pinder, R. (1992) Coherence and incoherence: Doctors' and patients' perspectives on the diagnosis of Parkinson's disease, *Sociology of Health and Illness*, 14(1), 1–22.

Qureshi, B. (1991) Traditions of ethnic minority groups. In A. Squires (ed.) *Multicultural Health Care and Rehabilitation*. London, Edward Arnold and Age Concern England, pp. 59–68.

Qureshi, H. (1990) Social support In S.M. Peace (ed.) *Researching Social Gerontology: Concepts, Methods and Issues*, London, Sage, pp. 32–45.

Qureshi, H. and Walker, A. (1989) *The Caring Relationship: Elderly People and their Families*, London, Macmillan.

Radley, A. (1989) Style, discourse and constraint in adjustment to chronic illness, *Sociology of Health and Illness*, 11, 231–52.

Rakowski, W. (1979) Future Time Perspective in Later Adulthood: Review and Research Directions. *Experimental Ageing Research*, 5: 43–88.

Rakowski W. and Hickey, T. (1980) Later life health behavior, *Research on Aging*, 2(3), September, 283–308.

Richardson, A. and Goodman, M. (1983) *Self–Help and Health: Mutual Aid for Modern Problems*. London: Martin Robertson.

Riley, J.C. (1987) *The Eighteenth Century Campaign to Avoid Disease*. New York, St Martin.

Roberts, H. (1985) *The Patient Patients*. London, Pandora Press.

Robertson, J. (1993) Possible futures for work. In A. Beattie, M. Gott, L. Jones and M. Sidell (eds) *Health and Wellbeing: A Reader*. London, Macmillan, pp. 287–96.

Rogers, A., Rogers, R.G. and Belanger, A. (1990) Longer life but worse health? Measurement and dynamics, *The Gerontologist*, 30(5), 640–9.

Roos, N.P. and Shapiro, E. (1981) The Manitoba longitudinal study on ageing: Preliminary findings on health care utilisation by the elderly, *Medical Care*, 19, 6.

Rotter, J.B. (1966) 'Generalised expectancies for internal versus external control reinforcement'. *Psychological Monographs*, 80: 1.
Royal College of General Practitioners/OPCS and DHSS (1986) *Morbidity Statistics from General Practice*. 3rd National Study 1981/2. London, HMSO.
Sarason, I. and Sarason, B. (eds) (1985) *Social Support: Theory, Research and Applications*. Dordrecht, The Netherlands, Nijhoff.
Scheiber, G.J. and Poullier, J.P. (1987) Recent trends in international health care spending, *Health Affairs*, 4, 105–12.
Schroder, F. (1993) Prostate cancer: to screen or not to screen? *British Medical Journal* 206, 13 February, 407–8.
Scrutton, S. (1992) *Ageing, Healthy and in Control*. London, Chapman Hall.
Segal, L. (1983) *What Is To Be Done About the Family?* Harmondsworth, Penguin.
Seligman, M.E.P. (1975) *Helplessness: on Depression Development and Death*. San Francisco, Freeman.
Shapiro, J. (ed.) (1989) *Ourselves Growing Older: Women Aging with Knowledge and Power*. London, Fontana.
Sharma, U. (1990) Using alternative therapies: Marginal medicine and central concerns. In P. Abbott and G. Payne (eds) *New Directions in the Sociology of Health*, London, Falmer Press, pp. 127–39.
Sidell, M. (1986) 'Coping with confusion: The experience of sixty elderly people and their carers', unpublished PhD thesis, Norwich, University of East Anglia.
Sidell, M. (1991) *Gender Differences in the Health of Older People*. Research report, Department of Health and Social Welfare, Milton Keynes, Open University.
Sidell, M. (1992) The relationship of elderly women to their doctors. In J. George and S. Ebrahim (eds) *Health Care for Older Women*, Oxford, Oxford University Press, pp. 179–96.
Sidell, M. (1993) Death, dying and bereavement. In J. Bond, P. Coleman and S. Peace (eds) *Ageing in Society: an introduction to social gerontology*. 2nd Edn, London, Sage, pp. 151–79.
Sixsmith, A.J. (1986) Independence and home in later life. In C. Phillipson, M. Bernard and P. Strang (eds) *Dependency and Interdependency in Old Age – Theoretical Perspectives and Policy Alternatives*. London, Croom Helm, pp. 338–47.
Smith, R. (1992) Osteoporosis. In J. George and S. Ebrahim (eds) *Health Care for Older Women*. Oxford, Oxford University Press, pp. 109–29.
Social Science and Medicine (1989) Special Issue on Self-care, 29(2).
Squires, A. (ed.) (1991) *Multicultural Health Care and Rehabilitation of Older People*. London, Edward Arnold and Age Concern England.
Stainton-Rogers, W. (1991) *Explaining Health and Illness: An Exploration of Diversity*. Hemel Hempstead, Harvester.
Stainton-Rogers, W. (1993) From Psychometric scales to cultural perspectives. In A. Beattie, M. Gott, L. Jones and M. Sidell (eds) *Health and Well-being: A Reader*. London: Macmillan.
Strauss, A. (1975) *Chronic Illness and the Quality of Life*. St Louis, Mosby.
Stevens, R. (1990) Humanistic Psychology. In I. Roth (ed.) *Introduction to Psychology*. Milton Keynes, Open University and Lawrence Erlbaum Associates.
Tardy, C.H. (1985) Social support measurement, *American Journal of Community Psychology*, 13, 187–202.
Taylor, R. and Ford, G. (1981) Lifestyle and ageing: Three traditions in lifestyle research, *Ageing and Society*, 1, 329.
Taylor, R. and Ford, G. (1983) Inequalities in old age: An examination of age, sex and class differences in a sample of community elderly, *Aging and Society*, 3(2), 182–208.
Taylor, R. et al. (1983) *The Elderly at Risk: A Critical Review of Problems and Progress in Screening and Case-finding*, Research Perspectives No. 6. London, Age Concern England.

Thoits, P.A. (1982) Conceptual, methodological and theoretical problems in studying social support as a buffer against life stress, *Journal of Health and Social Behaviour* 23, 145.

Thompson, P., Itzin, C. and Abendstein, M. (1990) *I Don't Feel Old – The Experience of Later Life*. Oxford, Oxford University Press.

Tilston, J. and Williams, J. (1992) 'Everyone wants to go to heaven but nobody wants to die'. Screening women over 75 – a health promotion approach. In J. George and S. Ebrahim (eds) *Health Care for Older Women*. Oxford, Oxford University Press, pp. 205–21.

Titterton, M. (1992) Managing threats to welfare: the search for a new paradigm of welfare, *Journal of Social Policy*, 21(1), 1–23.

Townsend, P. (1981) The structured dependency of the elderly: a creation of social policy in the 20th century, *Ageing and Society*, 1(1), 5–28.

Townsend, P. and Davidson, N. (eds) (1986) *Inequalities in Health: The Black Report*. Harmondsworth, Penguin.

Tulloch, A.J. and Moore, V. (1979) A randomised controlled trial of geriatric screening and surveillance in general practice, *Journal of the Royal College of General Practitioners*, 29.

Twycross, R.G. (1993) Assisted Death: A Reply, In D. Dickenson and M. Johnson (eds) *Death, Dying and Bereavement*. London, Sage.

Ungerson, C. (1983) Why do women care? In J. Finch and D. Groves (eds) *A Labour of Love*. London, Routledge and Kegan Paul.

Vachon, M.L.S. and Stylianos, S.K. (1988) The role of social support in bereavement, *Journal of Social Issues*, 44(3), 175–90.

Veiel, H.O.F. (1985) Dimensions of social support: A conceptual framework for research, *Social Psychiatry*, 20, 156–62.

Verbrugge, L.M. (1976) Sex differentials in morbidity and mortality in the United States, *Social Biology*, 23, 276–96.

Verbrugge, L.M. (1978) Sex and gender in health and medicine, *Social Science and Medicine*, 12, 329–33.

Verbrugge, L.M. (1983) Women and men: Mortality and health of older people. In M.W. Riley, B.B. Hess, and K. Bond (eds) *Ageing in Society: Selected Reviews of Recent Research*. Hillsdale, NJ, Laurence Erlbaum.

Verbrugge, L.M. (1984) Longer life but worsening health? Trends in health and mortality of middle-aged and older persons. *Milbank Memorial Fund Quarterly/Health and Society*, 62(3), 475–519.

Verbrugge, L.M. (1989). Gender, aging and health. In K.S. Markides (ed.) *Aging and Health: Perspectives on Gender, Race, Ethnicity, and Class*. Newbury Park, CA, Sage Publications Inc., pp. 23–78.

Victor, C. (1991) *Health and Health Care in Later Life*. Milton Keynes, Open University Press.

Waldron, I. (1976) Why do women live longer than men? *Journal of Human Stress*, 2, 2–13.

Waldron, I. (1982) Analysis of causes of sex differences in mortality and morbidity. In W.R. Gove and G.R. Carpenter (eds) *The Fundamental Connection Between Nature and Nurture*. Lexington, MA, Lexington Books, pp. 69–116.

Waldron, I. (1983) Sex differences in illness incidence, prognosis and mortality: Issues and evidence, *Social Science and Medicine*, 17, 1107–23.

Walker, A. (1993) Community Care Policy: from consensus to conflict, In J. Bornat, C. Pereira, D. Pilgrim and F. Williams (eds) *Community Care: A Reader*. London, Macmillan, pp. 204–226.

Wallen, J. (1979) Physician stereotyping about female health and illness: A study of patient's sex and the information process during medical interviews, *Women and Health*, 4, 135–45.

Weale, A. (1988) *Cost and Choice in Health Care: The Ethical Dimension*. London, King Edward's Hospital Fund for London.
Weiss, P. (1974) The provisions of social relationships, In Z. Rubin, *Doing unto others*. Englewood Cliffs, NJ, Prentice Hall.
Wells, N. and Freer, C. (eds) (1988) *The Ageing Population: Burden or Challenge?* London, Macmillan.
Wenger, G.C. (1984) *The Supportive Network: Coping with Old Age*. London, Allen and Unwin.
Wenger, G.C. (1988) *Old People's Health and Experience of the Caring Services: Accounts from Rural Communities in North Wales*. Liverpool, Liverpool University Press.
Whelan, C. (1993) The role of social support in mediating the psychological consequences of economic stress, *Sociology of Health and Illness*, 15(1), 86–101.
Whitehead, M. (1987) *The Health Divide*. Harmondsworth, Penguin.
Widgery, D. (1991) *Some Lives: A GP's East End*. London, Sinclair-Stevenson.
Wiener, C. (1975) The burden of rheumatoid arthritis: tolerating the uncertainty. In A. Strauss (ed.) *Chronic Illness and the Quality of Life*. St Louis, Mosby.
Wilkin, D. and Hughes, B. (1986) The elderly and the health services. In C. Phillipson and A. Walker (eds) *Ageing and Social Policy: A Critical Assessment*. Aldershot, Gower.
Williams, E.I. and Wilkin, D. (1988) GP care of the elderly: There's a fly in the ointment, *Geriatric Medicine*, May, 35–40.
Williams, F. (1992) 'Structural inequalities and the management of personal welfare: a selective literature review and assessment'. Unpublished discussion paper.
Williams, G. (1984) The genesis of chronic illness: Narrative reconstruction, *Sociology of Health and Illness*, 6, 174–200.
Williams, G. (1989) Hope for the humblest? The role of self-help in chronic illness: The case of ankylosing spondylitis, *Sociology of Health and Illness*, 11, 135–59.
Williams, R.G.A. (1983) Concepts of health: An analysis of lay logic, *Sociology*, 17, 185–204.
Williams, R.G.A. (1990) *The Protestant Legacy: Attitudes to Death and Illness Among Older Aberdonians*. Oxford, Oxford University Press.
Williamson, J., Stokoe, I.H. and Gray, S. et al. (1964) Old people at home: Their unreported needs. *Lancet* 23 May.
World Health Organization (WHO) (1980) *International Classification of Impairments, Disabilities and Handicaps*. Geneva, WHO.
World Health Organization (WHO) (1981) *Health for All by the Year 2000*. Geneva, WHO
World Health Organization (WHO) (1985) *Targets for health for all, 2000*, Copenhagen, World Health Organization.
World Health Organization Regional Office for Europe (1984) *Health promotion: a discussion document on the concept and principles*. Copenhagen, World Health Organization.
World Health Organization (1987) *World Health Statistics*. Geneva, WHO.
Wright, S. (1990) *My Patient – My Nurse*. London, Scutari Press.

Index

Aakster, C., 126
Acheson Report, 159
acute health problems, 41
Afro-Caribbean older people, 29, 45, 122, 143, 160
ageist, xvi, 32, 142, 162, 163
alternative therapy, 12, 13, 14, 126, 127
Anderson, R., 57, 58, 65, 69
Antonovsky, A., xvii, 14, 15, 16, 17, 57, 58, 61, 69, 70, 85, 86, 87, 105, 108, 130
Arber, S., xvi, 40, 47, 130, 132, 133, 134, 135, 144, 145
Ashton, J., 11, 12, 161, 162
Asian older people, 29, 45, 122, 125, 143, 157, 160

Baltes, M. M., 162
Barthel Index of ADL, 62
Beattie, A., xvii, 5, 6, 7, 8, 159
biomedical, xviii
  account, 3, 4, 6, 7
  model, 10, 11, 33
  tradition, 49, 57
biomedicine, 4, 6, 7, 8, 10, 11, 12, 13, 14, 126
Black Report, The, 9, 12, 14
Blakemore, K., xvi, 45, 66, 124, 125, 130, 143
Blaxter, M., 3, 4, 19, 20, 23, 24, 25, 27, 29, 30, 57, 58, 60, 62, 122

Boneham, M., xvi, 45, 124, 125, 143
Bosanquet, N., 118, 120
British Geriatric Society, 9, 10
Brown, G., 16, 131, 138
Burns, B., 41, 125
Bury, M., xv, 51, 57, 58, 59, 60, 61, 65, 67, 68, 69
Bytheway, B., xv, 142, 145

Calnan, M., 19, 20
Centre for Health in Retirement Education, 156
Chadwick, E., 6
Charmaz, K., 57, 58, 61, 62, 63, 65, 66, 69
chronic illness, xvi, xvii, 7, 15, 16, 24, 25, 41–7, 52, 53, 54, 57, 89, 130, 133, 148, 152, 162, 163
Cohen, S., 138, 139, 140
Coleman, P., 16, 137
Colerick, E., 16, 137, 138, 156
Collectivism, 129, 131, 146, 147, 150
Community Care, xiv, 115–18, 145, 146
  see also NHS and Community Care Act
complementary therapy, see alternative therapy
concepts of illness, 20, 21
Coni, N., xiii, 132
Coppard, L. C., 128
Cornwell, J., 3, 19, 20, 25, 28, 29, 51, 53
Coward, R., 14

Index

Cox, B. D., 18, 25

Dalley, G., 145, 146
Dant, T., 8, 115
Davidson, N., 7, 9, 12, 14, 130
Davison, C., 22
Dean, K., 127, 128
dependency, 60, 142, 146
  structured, 142
DHSS, 47, 48
disability, xv, xvii, 7, 15, 16, 24, 41–7, 52, 53, 57–9, 130, 133, 162, 163
Donovan, J., 29
Doyal, L., 111, 112
Draper, P., 158
Dubos, R., 7, 15

Ebrahim, S., xv, 45, 66, 122
Equal Opportunities Commission (EOC), 145
Erikson, E., 4, 5, 6, 27, 93, 105
euthanasia, 151, 152
Evers, H., 52, 113

Fennell, G., 66, 70
Finch, J., 144
Fletcher, A., 114
Ford, G., 47, 115, 122, 133, 143
Freud, 4
friendship, 140–2
Fries, J. F., xv, 40, 162

Gearing, B., 51, 81, 115
General Health Questionnaire (GHQ), 62
General Household Survey (GHS), 40, 41, 42, 43, 46, 51, 52, 53, 121, 134, 144
General Practitioner
  satisfaction with, 123
  use of, 121, 122
Gilbert, N., 144, 145
Ginn, J., xvi, 40, 47, 130, 132, 133, 134, 135
Goffman, E., 63
Groves, D., 144
Gunaratnam, Y., 66, 143, 144

Harris, T., 16, 131, 138
Hart, N., 8, 9, 11
health behaviours, 21
Health Education Council (HEC), 156
Health and Lifestyles Survey (HLS), 18, 19, 22, 23, 24, 27, 28, 44, 45, 50, 51, 52

Health Locus of Control, 16, 21
health promotion, xvi, 22, 154, 155, 158, 160, 161, 162
healthism, 162, 163
Henwood, M., 114, 144
Herzlich, C., 19, 20, 29, 31, 87
Hickey, T., 23, 127
holism, 6, 12, 13
holistic, 3, 6, 7, 8, 10
  account, 12, 13, 29, 33, 49, 114, 115, 126, 127
Hormone Replacement Therapy, 153
hospital care, 112, 113

illness behaviour, 29
individualism, 129, 131, 135, 147
informal carers, 105, 117, 143–7
Isaacs, B., 104
Itzin, C., 31, 32, 51, 52

Jamieson, A., 111, 112
Jerrome, D., 140–2
Johnson, M., 142, 154, 156, 158
Jones, L., xvii, 7, 159

Kitwood, T., 105, 106
Kobasa, S. C., 16, 131, 135, 136

Lazarus, R. S., 131, 135, 136
Lewis, M., xvi, 38, 51

MacIntyre, S., xiv, 112, 115
Maddi, S. R., 16, 131, 135, 136
Martin, J., 43, 44
Maslow, A., 6, 27, 105
medical model of health, 7, 32, 33, 89, 150, 153
Meltzer, H., 43, 44
mental health, 4
  illness, xvii, 40, 47–9
  malaise, 90–108
morbidity, 29, 33, 40–7, 51, 122
  compression of, xv, xvi, 162
  data, xvii, 8
  statistics, xv, 40
mortality, 9, 33–40, 119
  data, 8
  rectangularisation of, xv, 38
  statistics, 35, 39
Murphy, E., 16, 51, 90, 105, 139, 142

Nathanson, C. A., xvi, 51

178 Index

National Health Services (NHS), 6, 10, 11, 71, 79, 111–26, 127
  and Community Care Act, 115, 117, 152, 153
Norman, A., 45, 130

Office of Population Censuses and Surveys (OPCS), 34, 36, 38, 39, 41, 42, 43, 59, 119, 123

Passant, H., 127
Paterson, L., 19, 24, 25, 27, 29, 30, 58, 122
pathogenic paradigm, xvii, 14, 15, 32
phenomenology, 8
Phillipson, C., 41, 125, 155, 160
Pill, R., 21, 22
Pinder, R., 57, 58, 60, 65, 69
positivism, 8, 10
primary healthcare, 113–15
Public Health Movement, The, 6
  new, 12, 159

QALY, 150, 151
Qureshi, H., 117, 138, 139, 145

Radley, A., 57, 68
Reichert, M., 162
Robertson, J., 148, 149, 154, 161
Rose, H., 146
Rotter, J. B., 16
Royal College of General Practitioners, 42, 49, 121, 122
Royal College of Physicians, 9, 10

Salience of Lifestyle Index (SLI), 121
salutogenic paradigm, xvii, 16, 32, 70
screening, 114
Scrutton, S., 126
self-assessed health, 51–3
self-health care, 127–9
self-reported symptoms, 49
Seligman, M. E. P., 136

Sense of Coherence (SOC), 16, 17, 58, 61, 69, 85, 86, 87, 105
Seymour, H., 11, 12, 161, 162
social isolation, 65, 89, 140
social model of health, 7, 49, 114, 115, 158
social support, xiii, 89–106, 108, 129, 138–47
Stainton-Rogers, W., 3, 19, 21
Stott, N. C. H., 21, 22
Strauss, A., 57, 65, 67, 68, 69
sympatricity, 4, 7

Taylor, R., 47, 115, 122, 133, 143
Thompson, P., 31, 32, 51, 52
Tilston, J., 157
Titterton, M., 135
Townsend, P., 7, 9, 12, 14, 130, 142

Vachon, M. L. S., 138
Verbrugge, L. M., xvi, 35, 38, 41
victim blaming, 14, 158, 161
Victor, C., xvi, 51, 119, 132

Waldron, I., 35
Walker, A., 116, 117, 145
Weale, A., 151, 152
Wenger, C., 29, 31, 52, 53, 58, 120, 123, 124, 145
Whelan, C., 139
Whitehead, M., 7, 12, 34, 35, 130
WHO, 3, 4, 8, 10, 37, 54, 128, 154, 155, 158, 160, 161
Widgery, D., 132, 133
Wiener, C., 66, 67, 69
Wilkin, D., 112, 113
Williams, E. I., 113
Williams, F., 135
Williams, G., 57, 60, 129
Williams, J., 157
Williams, R. G. A., 19, 20, 30, 31, 52, 58, 62, 87, 89

AGE, RACE AND ETHNICITY
A COMPARATIVE APPROACH

Ken Blakemore and Margaret Boneham

This is the first definitive study of ageing among black and Asian people in Britain. Until now, debates on race relations have tended to ignore the 'greying' of Britain's minority communities. Equally, ageing studies have lacked a focus on the challenging realities of a multi-racial society and of racial discrimination. In this wide-ranging and questioning book, the authors combine original research with the results of over a decade of community studies of age and race. They give a comprehensive overview of the British context of 'minority ageing', comparing it with that of other societies such as the USA and Australia. They show the range and variety of patterns of ageing in the Asian and Afro-Caribbean communities, illustrated by personal life histories, and there are substantial chapters on the challenges to be faced by the health and social services. This book will be essential reading, both for 'reflective practitioners' and for anyone concerned with new developments in the fields of ageing, race relations, sociology and social policy.

> This is an important reference book for practitioners, professionals, gerontologists and students who want to gain an understanding of the realities, complexities and implications of providing comprehensive quality services for black and ethnic minority elders... The authors present significant social and demographic background studies from a range of sources... Professionals and students will find this book valuable as a research tool and for general information and further exploration of the subject.
>
> I hope *Age, Race and Ethnicity: A Comparative Approach* finds its way into all good bookshops, social service libraries and every social policy and gerontology reading list. It is value for money.
>
> *(Care Weekly)*

Contents
Introduction – Research, understanding and action – Comparative perspectives – Double jeopardy? – The Afro-Caribbean's experience – The Asians' experiences – Health, illness and health services – Welfare and social services – Conclusion – Bibliography – Index.

176pp   0 335 19086 3 (Paperback)   0 335 19234 3 (Hardback)

REMINISCENCE REVIEWED
PERSPECTIVES, EVALUATIONS, ACHIEVEMENTS

Joanna Bornat (ed.)

Since the 1980s the use of reminiscence and recall in caring situations has enjoyed immense popularity and now plays a central part in working with older people. Despite this fact, there is no single volume which critically evaluates the practice, its outcomes and achievements. This book aims to fill that gap by bringing together for the first time work by leading psychologists, gerontologists, social workers, nurses and community workers – who have first-hand experience of reminiscence work. The contributors take a critical overview of the field, standing back to look at their own and others' practice. They reflect on the processes involved in specific contexts and suggest ways of developing more sensitive approaches in an area of work which has seen much activity, but little reflection and evaluation. The book includes descriptions of work in hospitals, schools and a variety of community settings and will be invaluable to a wide range of students and practitioners in health, social care and adult education.

Contents
Introduction – Reminiscence within the study of ageing: The social significance of story – What splendour, it all coheres: Life-review therapy with older people – An interesting confusion: What can we do with reminiscence groupwork? – What can reminiscence contribute to people with dementia? – Reminiscence reviewed: A discourse analytic perspective – Beyond anti-ageism: Reminiscence groups and the development of anti-discriminatory social work education and practice – A fair hearing: Life-review in a hospital setting – 'I got put away': Group-based reminiscence with people with learning difficulties – Dramatizing reminiscences – Turning talking into writing – Arthos Wales: Working in hospitals – References – Index.

Contributors
John Adams, Dorothy Atkinson, Mike Bender, Joanna Bornat, Kevin Buchanan, Peter Coleman, Patricia Duffin, Jeffrey Garland, Faith Gibson, John Harris, Tom Hopkins, Rosie Mere, David Middleton, Pam Schweitzer.

160pp   0 335 19041 3 (Paperback)   0 335 19042 1 (Hardback)